Self-Assessment Colour Review of

Paediatric Nursing and Child Health

Judith Hunter MBE RGN, RSCN, RCNT Cert Ed,
MA, BSc (Hons)
Royal Victoria Infirmary
Newcastle upon Tyne
Tyne & Wear, UK

Veronica D. Feeg PhD, RN, FAAN
George Mason University
Fairfax, Virginia, USA

Marion E. Broome PhD, RN, FAAN
University of Alabama at Birmingham
Birmingham, Alabama, USA

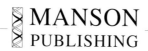
MANSON
PUBLISHING

Self-Assessment Colour Review of Paediatric Nursing and Child Health
Judith Hunter, Veronica D. Feeg and Marion E. Broome
ISBN: 1–874545–97–9

This edition reissued in 2003

Copyright © 2000, 2003 Manson Publishing Ltd

A CIP catalogue record for this book is available from the British Library.

For full details of all Manson Publishing Ltd titles please write to:
Manson Publishing Ltd, 73 Corringham Road, London NW11 7DL, UK.

Tel: +44(0)20 8905 5150
Fax: +44(0)20 8201 9233

Email: manson@man-pub.demon.co.uk
Website: www.manson-publishing.co.uk

Printed and bound in Spain and the United Kingdom

Preface

Today's nurse is confronted daily with clinical challenges that call upon a wide array of technology-based knowledge and skills. In addition to working from a substantive scientific foundation for assessment and management of pediatric clinical conditions, the children's nurse today also must be well versed in all aspects of the health care of children over the developmental periods of infancy, childhood, and adolescence. These aspects include the health promotion and disease prevention concerns that the nurse may address in community settings, as well as the acute care, critical care, and chronic care needs of sick children in hospitals. This book provides nurses with a review of questions and answers that covers an assortment of topics, conditions, and care roles in pediatric settings in the USA and UK.

The task of assembling a range of questions related to the multiple aspects of pediatric nursing practice was tackled by the editors using a conceptual framework that is rooted in the nursing process, assessment of common childhood conditions and management of clinical care. While the nurse needs to use nursing skills of observation and communication to assess the signs and symptoms of diseases, the nurse may not be the disease diagnostician in the process. Rather, the nursing role as a member of an interdisciplinary team requires that the nurse has a full understanding of the disease process and recommended therapies while providing care to the child and family in any given health care situation.

A matrix of developmental periods subdivided by the aspects of acute/critical conditions, chronic conditions, and health promotion or disease prevention was developed and related to a list of diseases and childhood problems. From the matrix, a variety of question areas were generated such that the clinical problems presented in the topics would be in question format relative to some aspect of nursing care. Many contributors with specialized expertise in pediatric nursing were solicited from the USA and the UK. Their questions and answers in this book reflect the matrix of developmental periods of childhood and adolescence, and mirror the wide variety of clinical care settings in which nurses from both countries work.

All nurses working today in child or family settings would benefit by periodically stretching their repertoire of knowledge over the expanse of information requisite in general pediatric practice. This book will help clinicians to review disease-related content while problem-solving clinical situations that sample the massive database in pediatric nursing practice.

Judith Hunter
Veronica D. Feeg
Marion E. Broome

Contributors

MaryAnn Alexander, MS, RN
University Orthopedics,
Rush-Presbyterian-St Luke's Medical
Center, Chicago, Illinois, USA

Carole C. Atkinson, MS, RNC, PNP
Children's Hospital, Boston,
Massachusetts, USA

Patricia Ann Bailey, MSN, RN
La Rabida Children's Hospital,
Chicago, Illinois, USA

Rosemary Briars, ND, RN, CPNP, CDE
La Rabida Children's Hospital
Chicago, Illinois, USA

Marion E. Broome, PhD, RN, FAAN
Professor and Associate Dean of Research,
University of Alabama at Birmingham,
Birmingham, Alabama, USA

Carol A. Chesley, RN, CPNP
University of Wisconsin–Milwaukee,
Milwaukee, Wisconsin, USA

Janice Clarke, RGN, RSCN
Royal Victoria Infirmary,
Newcastle upon Tyne,
Tyne & Wear, UK

Amy Delaney, MSN, RN, CPNP
Children's Hospital, Boston,
Massachusetts, USA

Laura S. Deery, MS, RNC
Hospital for Sick Children,
Washington DC, USA

Jane Devine, MS, RN, CPNP
Hospital for Sick Children,
Washington DC, USA

Rachel DiFazio, PNP-O
Children's Hospital, Boston,
Massachusetts, USA

Veronica D. Feeg, PhD, RN, FAAN
Professor of Nursing,
George Mason University,
Fairfax, Virginia, USA

MaryEllen Freeman, MSN, RN
Children's Hospital of Wisconsin,
Milwaukee, Wisconsin, USA

Linda L. Gehring, MS, RNCS, FNP
University of Wisconsin–Milwaukee,
Milwaukee, Wisconsin, USA

Julie Guest, RGN, RN Dip, BSc (Hons)
Royal Victoria Infirmary,
Newcastle upon Tyne,
Tyne & Wear, UK

Judith Hunter, RGN, RSCN, RCNT
Cert Ed, MA, BSc (Hons)
Royal Victoria Infirmary
Newcastle upon Tyne,
Tyne & Wear, UK

Martha Kliebenstein, MSN, RN
Olsen Health Services,
Milwaukee, Wisconsin, USA

Colleen McCann, MN, RN CAPNP
Children's Hospital of Wisconsin,
Milwaukee, Wisconsin, USA

Heather A. LoRe, MSN, RNC
Children's Hospital, Boston,
Massachusetts, USA

James A. Metcalf, PhD
Professor
College of Nursing and Health Science,
George Mason University,
Fairfax, Virginia, USA

Karen Nugent-Brennan, BSN, RN
Children's Hospital, Boston,
Massachusetts, USA

Patricia Ring, MSN, RN
Children's Hospital of Wisconsin,
Milwaukee, Wisconsin, USA

Lucia Russell, RGN, RSCN, CCN,
DPSN (DN), BSc (Hons)
Newcastle upon Tyne Hospitals NHS
Trust, Newcastle upon Tyne,
Tyne & Wear, UK

Sharon K. Schroeder, MSN, CPNP
Children's Hospital of Wisconsin,
Milwaukee, Wisconsin, USA

Judith S. Shaw, MPH, RN
Massachusetts Poison Control System,
Boston, Massachusetts, USA

Donna Shelly, MS, RN
Georgetown University Child
Development Center,
Washington DC, USA

Anastasia M. Snelling, PhD, RD
American University,
Washington DC, USA

Julia Snethen, PhD, RN
University of Wisconsin–Milwaukee
Milwaukee, Wisconsin, USA

Sheila Lenihan Walsh, MA, RNC
Overlook Hospital, Summit,
New Jersey, USA

Jeni Wincek, MSN, RN
Goshen General Hospital, Goshen,
Indiana, USA

Susan Vernon, RGN, RSCN, BA (Hons)
University of Newcastle upon Tyne,
Newcastle upon Tyne,
Tyne & Wear, UK

Reviewers

Megan M. Davis, DNSc, RN
Loudoun County Public Schools,
Sterling, Virginia, USA

Kathleen Ryan Kuntz, MSN, RN,
CRRN, CLCP
Jamison, Pennsylvania, USA

Picture acknowledgements

1, 5 Photographs from personal collection. Source unknown.

9, 14 Courtesy of St John's Institute of Dermatology.

10 Courtesy of J. Shaw.

12, 47, 95 Central Sheffield University Hospitals.

19 Used with permission, Eli Lilly and Company, 1998. All rights reserved.

20, 87 Photographs courtesy of Ildiko Kunos.

40, 112 Wellcome Trust Medical Photographic Library.

46 Extrophy of the bladder: reconstruction allows continence for the first time. Sui GENERIS. Milwaukee, WI: Children's Hospital of Wisconsin, Summer, 1997, pp. 22–24.

51 Extrophy of the bladder. Sui GENERIS. Milwaukee, WI: Children's Hospital of Wisconsin, Summer, 1997, p. 25.

55 Redrawn from Peck, K. (1988) Intraosseous infusion. *Pediatric Nursing*, **14**(4): 221–6.

56 Zitelli, B. and Davis, H. (1992). *Atlas of Pediatric Physical Diagnosis*, 2nd edn. Gower Medical Publishing, New York, pp. 3.14–3.15.

60 Courtesy of Ross Laboratories.

61 Adapted from Centers for Disease Control and Prevention (1993). 1993 sexually transmitted diseases. *Morbidity and Mortality Weekly Reports*, **42**(RR–14) 75–81.

64 Redrawn from Iazzetti, L. (1991). Dysrhythmias in the pediatric AIDS patient. *Pediatric Nursing*, **17**(1): 49–51.

68 Redrawn from an illustration courtesy of Thomas F. Plant MD.

69 Table 1: Language Development (adapted from Nicolosi, L., Harryman, E. and Kreshcck, J. (1989). *Terminology of Communication Disorders-Speech-Language-Hearing*, 3rd edition. Williams & Wilkins, Baltimore. [pp. 297–301].

70 Jennett, B. and Teasdale, G. (1977). Aspects of coma after severe head injury. *Lancet*, **1**(8017), 878–81.

74 Adapted from a diagram by Patsy S. Huff in Harbin, R. (1995). Female adolescent contraception. *Pediatric Nursing*, **21**(3): 221–6.

75 Redrawn from Curley, M.A. and Thompson, J.E. (1990). End-tidal CO_2 monitoring in critically ill infants and children. *Pediatric Nursing*, **16**(4): 397–403.

76 Redrawn from Iazzetti, L. (1991). Dysrhythmias in the pediatric AIDS patient. *Pediatric Nursing*, **17**(1): 49–51.

Abbreviations

AIDS   acquired immune deficiency syndrome
AMA   arm muscle area
ANC   absolute neutrophil count
AP   anteroposterior
APGAR   method of evaluating the well-being of a new-born infant by assigning a score to five parameters: heart rate, respiratory effort, muscle tone, reflex irritability, color
AV   arteriovenous
b.i.d.   *bis in die* (twice a day)
BLS   Basic Life Support
BMI   body mass index
BP   blood pressure
BPD   bronchopulmonary dysplasia
BUN   blood urea nitrogen
CBC   complete blood count
CDC   Centers for Disease Control and Prevention
CSF   cerebrospinal fluid
CT   computed tomography
DKA   diabetic ketoacidosis
DMSA   dimercaptosuccinic acid
DPT/HIB   diptheria, pertussis, tetanus, *Hemophilus influenzae* type B
DQ   developmental quotient
ECG (UK)   electrocardiogram
EDA (UK)   estimated date of arrival
EDC (US)   estimated date of confinement
EEG   electroencephalogram
EIA   exercise-induced asthma
EKG (US)   electrocardiogram
ESR   erythrocyte sedimentation rate
FAS   fetal alcohol syndrome
FEF_{25-75} forced expiratory flow between 25% and 75% vital capacity
FEV_1 forced expiratory volume in 1 second
FVC   forced vital capacity (maximum amount of air forcibly exhaled after maximum inhalation)

GCS   Glasgow Coma Scale
GI   gastrointestinal
HIB   *Hemophilus influenzae* type B
HIV   human immunodeficiency virus
ICU   Intensive Care Unit
IPV   inactivated polio vaccine
IQ   intelligence quotient
IVH   intraventricular hemorrhage
LFT   liver function test
MAC   mid-arm circumference
MDI   metered dose inhaler
MMR   measles, mumps, rubella
MRI   magnetic resonance imaging
NEC   necrotizing enterocolitis
NG   nasogastric
NPO   *nil per oris* (nothing by mouth)
OPV   oral polio vaccine
PE (tube)   pressure equalizing (tube)
PEFR   peak expiratory flow rate
PID   pelvic inflammatory disease
p.r.n.   *pro re nata* (as required)
PT   pro.time (prothrombin time)
PVC   premature ventricular contractions
PVL   periventricular leukomalacia
q.i.d.   *quater in die* (four times a day)
RN   reflux nephropathy
RSV   respiratory syncytial virus
SBE   subacute bacterial endocarditis
SBGM   self-blood glucose monitoring
SBS   shaken baby syndrome
SVT   supraventricular tachycardia
TENS   transcutaneous electrical nerve stimulation
t.i.d.   *ter in die* (three times a day)
TKAFO   thigh-knee-ankle-foot orthosis
TPN   total parenteral nutrition
URI   upper respiratory infection
UTI   urinary tract infection
VC   vital capacity
VUR   vesicouteric reflux
WBC   white blood cell
WPW   Wolff-Parkinson-White (syndrome)

Classification of cases

1 This infant (1) had been a 30-week, preterm baby who developed NEC and became critically ill within the first few weeks of life.

i. What are the possible etiologies of this condition?

ii. What are the clinical signs and mortality rate associated with this condition?

iii. What are the nursing interventions in early stages?

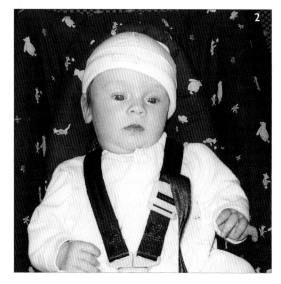

2 In the UK, about 100 children are killed each year as a result of car accidents in which they are passengers. Approximately 1,800 children are seriously injured and a further 9,000 will receive slight injuries as occupants of cars. Accident prevention is the best approach to reducing fatalities and serious injury.

i. How can car safety be improved (2)?

ii. What are the best types of car safety devices for children of different age groups?

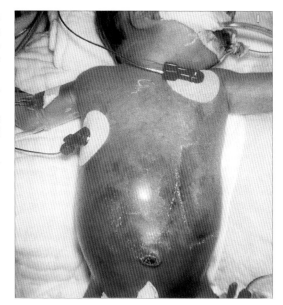

I & 2: Answers

1 i. NEC is a condition of diffuse, patchy necrosis of the mucosa or submucosa of the small and/or large bowel. The most common sites are the terminal ileum and colon. To date, there is no unifying theory regarding the pathogenesis of NEC, although major factors which seem to contribute include ischemic injury (including vasospasm), thrombosis or low flow states, selective vascular ischemia, or bacterial colonization enhanced by other conditions such as excess bacterial toxins. Other associated risk factors include prematurity and low birthweight, abruptio placenta, and hypertonic milk feedings.
ii. Abdominal distention with visible loops of bowel, increased gastric residuals, vomiting, bloody stools and/or NG aspirate, temperature instability, and abdominal distention resulting in shiny, reddened abdominal wall, apnea, and bradycardia. NEC is the major cause of death of newborns undergoing surgery, greater than all other congenital abnormalities of the GI tract combined, ranging from 20–75% depending on gestational age and other newborn conditions.
iii. In the early stages, or in suspected NEC, isolation, strict handwashing, and gowns and gloves should be used. Nursing interventions to support medical treatment include bowel decompression (NG to suction, measure, and replace), fluid and electrolyte restoration, antibiotics, monitoring abdominal girths frequently, assessing bowel sounds, no rectal temperatures taken, avoiding diapers, frequent turning, and prevention of skin breakdown.

2 i. The use of child restraints is a very important aspect in reducing the number of injuries in the event of an accident. The correct use of occupant restraint can reduce the rate of serious injury by 40–70% and fatalities by 50–90%. Restraints can prevent the child from either being thrown out of the vehicle or hitting hard objects in the period of rapid deceleration following impact.
ii. Safety devices for different age groups allowable in the UK:

Age/weight of child	Type of device	Where fitted
0–9 months (up to 10 kg [22 lb])	Infant carrier Carry cot in carry cot straps	Front or rear seat Rear seat placed sideways
6–9 months to 4 years (10–18 kg [22–40 lb])	Child safety seat	Front- or rear-facing seat
Young child (4–9 years) (18–36 kg [40–80 lb])	Booster seat with adult seat belt or 4-point harness	Front or rear seat
Older child (≥10 years)	Standard adult seat belt	Front or rear seat

Each country will have specific regulations about child car safety which should be strictly adhered to. For example, in the USA it is recommended that, whenever possible, child safety seats and infant carriers are always fitted in the rear seats; in cars with passenger airbags, children younger than 12 years cannot be seated in the front seat.

3 A 30-year-old father and his 10-year-old son are preparing to do a long distance run together. The father asks for advice about training for the event related to his and his son's heart rate.

i. What are the acceptable heart rates for pediatric populations during physical activity, and how do they differ from adults?

ii. What special considerations should be taken into account when recommending exercise for this father and son?

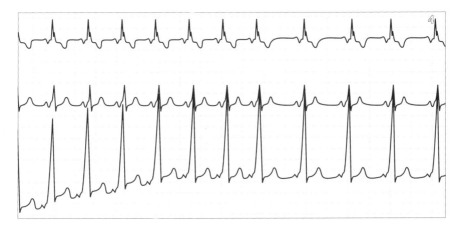

4 A 12-year-old female with no known illness presents to the Emergency Department with loss of consciousness. The incident occurred after a swim and lasted 20 minutes. Her symptoms started with chest pain radiating to her neck and head. She also felt dizzy and weak; she then vomited and fainted. She had no seizure-like activity. As she awakened, she experienced palpitations lasting approximately 10 minutes. She was transported via ambulance, an EKG (ECG) (4) was obtained and an intravenous line placed. She was diagnosed with WPW syndrome.

i. What EKG findings are characteristic of WPW?

ii. What are the clinical findings associated with WPW?

iii. What are the nursing interventions?

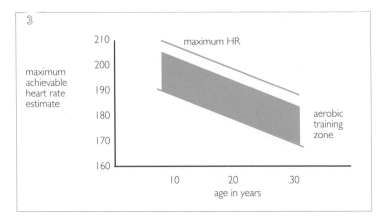

3 i. Maximal achievable heart rate tends to decrease with aging. Pediatric heart rates exceed adult heart rates both at rest and during exercise (3). The acceptable range of exercise heart rates for children does not differ from that of adults when given as a percentage of maximal achievable heart rate. However, since maximal achievable heart rate declines with age, children can be expected to achieve higher absolute heart rates than adults, especially during sustained aerobic exercise.

ii. Children should be encouraged to exercise at levels where they feel comfortable and experience no discomfort. They should be permitted, even encouraged, to reduce the intensity of their exercise, or to rest, whenever they so desire. Thermal control mechanisms may not be as effective so they should be especially sensitive to maintenance of adequate hydration and hyperthermia during sustained periods of physical activity.

4 i. WPW is characterized by a supraventricular tachydysrhythmia. The initial part of the QRS complex is slurred and is called the delta wave. It is the presence of this delta wave that confirms the diagnosis of WPW.

ii. Clinical findings or symptoms of WPW include syncope, faint feeling, heart racing or tachycardia, central chest pain, dizziness, and palpitations.

iii. Nursing interventions include symptomatic treatment. Bed-rest in semi-Fowler's position, oxygen via nasal cannula or nonrebreather apparatus, placement of a large-bore intravenous line, and an EKG are also indicated.

5 A mother giving a question-able prenatal history delivers a 2 kg (4 lb 6 oz) baby boy after a brief, uncomplicated labor. The delivery was one week before her calculated EDC (EDA), but the infant appeared much less mature than expected. His foot (**5a**) is compared with a normal term infant (**5b**). He has evidence of lanugo over his back and trunk. With his arm drawn across his chest until resistance

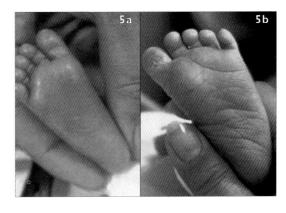

is met, his elbow extends beyond mid-line of his body (scarf sign). His ears have no cartilage.

i. What can the soles of the feet indicate about prematurity?
ii. What other clinical signs can assist in determining gestational age?
iii. What might the nurse conclude from these signs?

6 This young child (**6**) was healthy, with no obvious medical problems until the age of 16 months. After eating a biscuit containing peanut butter he rapidly developed blistered lips, an urticarial rash and a swollen face (angioedema). These symptoms all resolved within an hour. Six weeks later, he ate some pea-nut-butter on toast; on this occasion he began to retch and vomited. He became hoarse, and his breathing was labored with an audible wheeze. Severe angio-edema of his face was evident and he was immediately rushed to the Emergency Department.

i. What is an anaphylactic reaction?
ii. What are the physiologic changes that occur during anaphylaxis?

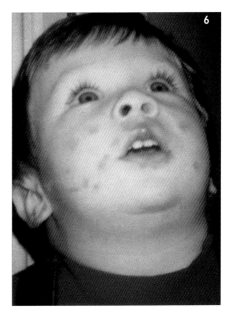

5 i. Plantar creases increase with gestational age and can verify prematurity. Assessed at the first 12 hours of life, plantar creases develop at the anterior portion first and proceed toward the heel. This infant shows no plantar creases on his thin, shiny skin.

ii. Preterm infants' skin is smooth and thin, red or pink, with visible veins. Below 28 weeks' gestation, infants have little or no lanugo, but at 28–30 weeks, lanugo is thickest. Lanugo slowly disappears from 31–40 weeks, and only small amounts are present at the shoulders and scapular areas at term. Premature infants before 34 weeks have no ear cartilage, develop slight curving of the upper pinna from 34–36 weeks, and at 40 weeks have two-thirds of the ear curved, that recoils to its original position if bent forward. The scarf sign (when the arm is drawn across the chest until resistance is met, and the elbow can reach past the mid-line of the body) indicates that the infant is less than 36 weeks. The genitalia of males, including the size and degree of rugation of the scrotum, indicate prematurity when the scrotum is small, has few rugae, and the testes are in the inguinal canal.

iii. This mother has not recalled accurately her last menstrual period, may have been irregular, or may not be giving a reliable history at all. This infant is clearly premature, probably well under 34 weeks, and should be monitored closely for developing respiratory or related complications.

6 i. Anaphylaxis is the medical term used to describe a severe, life-threatening systemic allergic reaction – the most extreme end of the allergy spectrum. It presents as a medical emergency and is the most urgent of clinical immunologic events. Anaphylactic shock requires immediate treatment. True anaphylaxis occurs when the body's immune system overreacts in response to the presence of a foreign body (allergen) which the body perceives as a threat. The whole body is affected during an anaphylactic reaction, usually within minutes of exposure to the allergen. Cases have been reported where a reaction has developed within an hour.

ii. An anaphylactic reaction is caused by a sudden release of chemical substances, including histamine, from the body's cells in the blood and tissues where they are stored. This outpouring is triggered by a reaction between the allergic type of antibody called IgE with the substance or allergen, resulting in anaphylactic shock. This mechanism is so sensitive that very minute quantities of an allergen are sufficient to cause a severe reaction. The released chemicals act on the blood vessels to cause swelling (angioedema) and low blood pressure, and on the lungs to cause wheezing and difficulty in breathing. This leads to respiratory obstruction, usually as a combined result of laryngeal edema, bronchial wall edema, and severe bronchospasm.

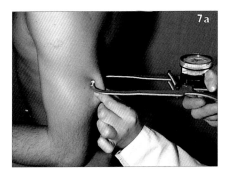
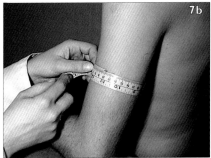

7 A young male adolescent, who was a refugee with questionable prior living and health conditions, was seen at the clinic for symptoms of fatigue and lethargy.
i. What two measurements are being taken on his arm (7a, b), and what can be calculated?
ii. What is the use of these measurements in patients?

8 This two-year-old female (8) arrives in the Emergency Department clearly un-well, with a fever and obvious discomfort when she passes urine. Her mother comments that the little girl's urine smells 'fishy'.
i. What is the possible diagnosis for this child?
ii. What immediate nursing interventions should be performed?
iii. What is the significance of UTI?

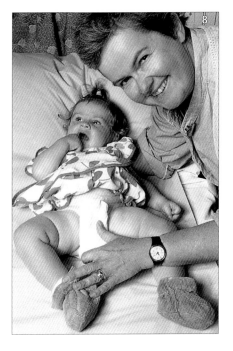

7 i. The triceps skinfold and MAC are being measured from the dominant arm and are used to determine indirectly the AMA. The AMA is a useful indication of the lean body mass and hence the skeletal protein reserves.

ii. Malnutrition is a possibility due to this patient's history. Since methods commonly used to assess nutritional status (i.e. dietary records) may be difficult to ascertain, this measure can provide valuable data on possible protein–energy malnourishment as a result of inadequate diet.

8 i. Discomfort on micturition may indicate that the child has vulval soreness; this may be due to irritation from the use of bubble bath or scented soap. The possibility of sexual abuse should also be considered. However, actual discomfort on micturition associated with fever and a 'fishy' or 'musty' smell usually indicates the presence of a UTI.

ii. Obtain a specimen of urine either by clean catch technique or using a urine collection pad. This will facilitate urgent microscopy, before starting an antibiotic, to establish the diagnosis of UTI.

Establish the child's temperature and implement appropriate cooling mechanisms, by the administration of an antipyretic drug and by sponging if necessary.

The child should be encouraged to drink plenty of fluids and, if it is considered necessary, an intravenous infusion may be administered.

iii. UTI in childhood is common, with approximately 3% of children affected, girls more than boys. UTI in conjunction with VUR can cause permanent renal damage. Some children develop renal scars that can extend with further bouts of UTI.

Hypertension develops in over 20% of patients with scars, and up to 10% may develop end-stage renal failure, often many years later. Scarring can only be initiated by UTIs in early childhood, and can occur very quickly after only a few days' infection.

Establishing a diagnosis of UTI can be very difficult in young children, as symptoms are often vague and nonspecific.

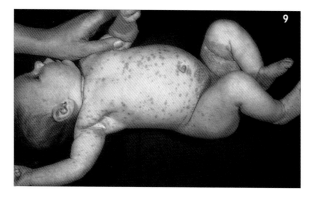

9 This infant (9) has been seen by the pediatrician for seborrheic dermatitis affecting the diaper (nappy) area.
i. How does the appearance and symptoms of seborrheic dermatitis differ from that of irritant dermatitis and atopic eczema in infancy?
ii. What therapies play a role in the treatment of seborrheic dermatitis affecting other areas of the infant, including the scalp, face, and upper trunk?

10 A 17-year-old female arrived home one afternoon after having a fight with her boyfriend at school. That evening her parents noted her to have repeated episodes of vomiting and was more quiet than usual. During the night she continued to vomit and by the next morning she was difficult to wake and very confused. Her parents immediately took her to the Emergency Department. There, her vital signs were normal except for sinus

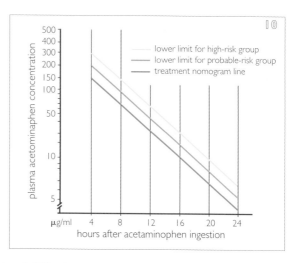

tachycardia. She was confused and difficult to arouse.
i. What is the probable diagnosis? What symptoms led you to this conclusion?
ii. What are the most common drugs ingested in an adolescent overdose?
iii. What is the standard treatment in an overdose and what does the graph (10) represent?
iv. What are the nursing interventions in a late presenting overdose?

9 i. The appearance contrasts with that of irritant dermatitis, which usually spares the groin flexures, and atopic eczema, which usually spares the moist diaper areas altogether. Additionally, seborrheic dermatitis, despite its raw appearance, is often asymptomatic, unlike the itch and discomfort of the others.
ii. Topical steroid therapy, antiseborrheic shampoos, and topical antifungal creams may all have a role to play in the treatment of severe cases, depending on the location on the body. Generally, however, mild conditions usually resolve fairly rapidly.

10 i. Intentional acetaminophen (paracetamol) overdose. Acetaminophen is the most common drug used in suicide attempts by adolescents. A presentation of an adolescent with an acute onset of vomiting and confusion should raise the suspicion of intentional overdose. Often in the early stages of acute overdose with acetaminophen the patient will be asymptomatic. As in this case, the only initial sign may be vomiting, with changes in mental status showing later. Blood and urine toxicology screens can confirm the diagnosis. A toxic dose is 7.5 g in adults and 150 mg/kg in children.
ii. Acetaminophen and cough and cold preparations are some of the most common drugs used by adolescents in both intentional and unintentional overdoses.
iii. Initial treatment of an acute acetaminophen ingestion includes gastric lavage and administration of activated charcoal with GI tract accelerant. In this example, as the patient presented 12–18 hours postingestion, and since acetaminophen is rapidly absorbed from the GI tract within 30–120 minutes, gastric lavage and GI decontamination will be of little benefit. Standard treatment after gastric decontamination includes the administration of the antidote N-acetylcysteine.

The graph (**10**) represents a nomogram for predicting which patients are at risk of developing hepatoxicity, the most serious complication of acetaminophen overdose. Toxicity is determined through plasma acetaminophen levels drawn at 4 hours post-ingestion. Levels prior to this time are inaccurate as complete absorption has not occurred.
iv. Vital sign monitoring, fluid rehydration, monitoring of plasma acetaminophen levels, PT and LFTs, and antiemetic and antidote administration. The known antidote, N-acetylcysteine, is successful in reversing the risk of acetaminophen-associated hepatitis, if administered within 24 hours postingestion.

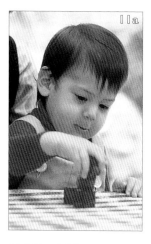 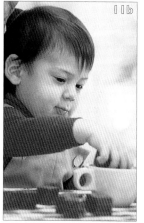 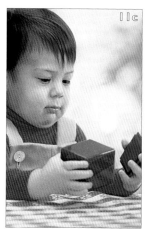

11 This child (**11a–c**) was tested for a possible developmental delay at 15 months with the Bayley Scales of Infant Development.
i. What can and cannot be learned from a developmental test?
ii. What cognitive and motor abilities are shown above?

12 A three-month-old male is admitted to the ward with bronchiolitis. His mother comments that he cries a lot, has difficulty feeding, and sleeps for short periods only, waking in the night screaming. He has an older sister who is two years old. The mother states that she is finding it difficult to cope with the children and that she is exhausted, having not slept properly since she became a mother. On examination, the infant appears to be well nourished, but does not smile. He follows objects, but does not reach out to touch them.

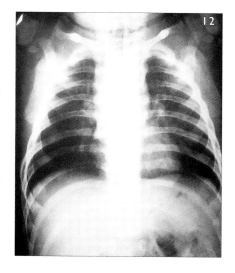

The infant has a chest X-ray (**12**) shortly after admission and it is noted that there are old, healed fractures of the posterior ribs.
i. Describe the nursing observations you would make regarding his physical care.
ii. What is the significance of the fractured ribs?
iii. What investigations should be undertaken now that there is suspicion of non-accidental injury?

11 & 12: Answers

11 i. Most developmental tests assess the infant or toddler's cognitive and fine/gross motor developmental abilities as compared with other infants or toddlers of the same age. They can reveal some areas of concern when the child cannot perform selective tasks that other children of the same chronological age can, even taking into account the infant's prematurity. The tests yield a DQ that should not be misinterpreted as an IQ or prediction of the child's future intellectual capability.

ii. In **11a**, the child is being asked to stack small cubes; this measures the child's fine motor coordination and ability to stay on a task over several repetitions. In **11b**, the child has to place cubes in a cup, which assesses his understanding of 'in the cup' along with elements from **11a**. In **11c**, the child is asked to 'find the bunny', which is a task that tests the child's 'object permanency' (i.e. the child's understanding that the object exists even if it is out of sight). The task also tests the child's ability to manipulate the box and look inside.

12 i. On admission, the child should be weighed and his length checked against the percentile charts to plot growth and development. It is important to obtain the weight of the child to assist in the prescribing of medication to ensure the correct dose per kilogram of body weight is administered.

Assessment of the child's overall appearance should be made, noting any bruising, rashes or unusual marks on the body. The respiratory rate and oxygen saturation should be closely monitored.

The nurse should remain nonjudgemental about possible child abuse, while observing family relationships and reactions to his sister.

ii. He has sustained fractures that are consistent with being shaken. The age of the fractures will determine the approximate date of the injury. The medical history will also be significant in enabling the medical team to find out what has happened to him in his short life. For example, the mother may recall him crying more than usual or recollect if he has appeared to be in pain.

iii. It is essential to carry out further investigations to exclude a physiologic explanation for the injuries, e.g. osteogenesis imperfecta:

- Full skeletal survey, repeated in 10–14 days to identify any old/new fractures.
- Ophthalmic examination to detect retinal hemorrhages – indicative of having been shaken.
- CT or MRI head scan to check for intracranial bleeding.
- Assessment of any external injuries is essential. These should also be photographed for future reference.
- All the investigations and assessments should be carried out by pediatric radiologists and pediatric ophthalmologists, ideally coordinated by a forensic pediatrician.

Motion	Right hip	Left hip
Flexion	90°	130°
Abduction	25°	50°
Adduction	15°	25°
Internal rotation	0°	25°
External rotation	15°	25°
Abductor strength	5+	4+

13 A five-year-old male has complained of left knee pain for the past month and his parents state they have noticed him limping. His knee examination is normal and X-rays taken of his knee by his primary care physician are normal. There is no history of trauma or fevers. He appears healthy and is developmentally appropriate for his age.
i. On which part of the physical examination should the nurse focus next?
    The hip examination reveals the above results.
ii. What diagnostic studies should be done?
iii. This child is diagnosed with Legg–Calvé–Perthes disease. Describe this condition, explain what types of patients are affected, and state what parents should be told about this disease.

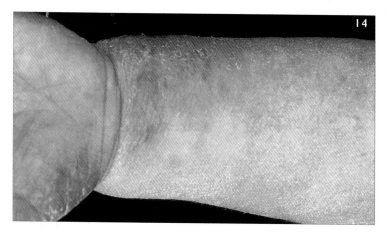

14 This child has atopic eczema (**14**) which had been inadequately treated.
i. What clinical signs indicate the chronicity of this type of exacerbation?
ii. What techniques are useful to treat moderate or severe eczema of any cause?
iii. What advice should this girl be given about bathing?

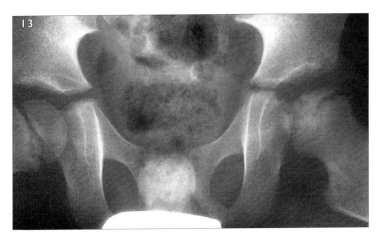

13 i. Since hip problems can be manifested by groin, thigh, or knee pain, the clinician should thoroughly examine this child's hips.

ii. The diagnostic study that should be obtained initially are X-rays of both hips (AP and lateral) (13).

iii. The parents should be told that this condition is avascular necrosis of the femoral head due to a disruption in the blood supply to the femoral head. The disease primarily affects children between the ages of three and eight years. Males are four times more likely to acquire this disease than females. One out of ten children have both hips affected. With time, the circulation will be remodeled and restored to the femoral head without any specific medical intervention. There are usually no residual functional problems.

14 i. The scratching and excoriation evidence on the forearm indicate the inadequacy of treatment and the discomfort the child must be experiencing. The skin is dry, red, and flaky and there are obvious signs of chronic scratching.

ii. In general, a topical corticosteroid can be used intensively for short periods of time. The corticosteroid should be applied and the area should then be occluded with polythene (i.e. self-adherent food-wrap) to prevent the loss of medication and enhance penetration into the skin. This technique helps retain lubrication of the area and prevents direct scratching.

iii. Children with eczema of any cause should avoid the use of soap and use emollients instead (including emulsifying ointment, aqueous cream, unperfumed bath oils) both in bathing and for regular topical application.

15 This one-year-old child (**15**) presented with progressive deformities and was diagnosed with Blount's disease.
i. What is the difference between physiologic bowing and Blount's disease?
ii. How is the diagnosis made, and when is treatment required?
iii. What treatment is needed, and how does the nurse support its success?

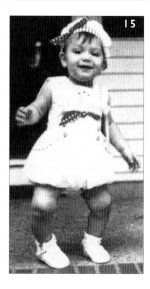

16 The introduction of solids into an infant's diet is a milestone in child development and a key moment in family life (**16**). Parents often make inquiries to the children's nurse, seeking information about the introduction of solids. What advice would you offer about the introduction of solids into an infant's diet?

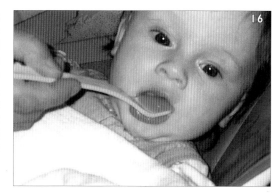

17 What should one of your primary assessments be in any child with a history of recurrent otitis media/chronic otitis media with effusion?

15–17: Answers

15 i. Physiologic bowing improves over time; however, children with Blount's disease get worse over time.
ii. From an X-ray of the hip, knee, and ankle. The leg is held so that the knee is in true AP position, even though the foot may be medially rotated; draw a line through the hip center to the ankle center. The abnormality requires intervention when the line passes through no bone at the knee.
iii. A TKAFO brace is used until correction is achieved. It must prevent lateral thrust, and must produce a mild corrective angular force at the knee. The flexed alignment of the brace must be gradually altered to correct the torsional abnormality, and the brace requires regular re-alignment and elongation to keep pace with growth. A simple prescription for TKAFO will fail. Mothers need education, encouragement, and support to use these cumbersome devices, especially during the toddler period. The nurse helps the mother to ensure compliance, which is critical to successful outcomes.

16 It is advisable to wait until an infant is three to four months old before considering the introduction of solids into the diet. If the baby appears still to be hungry following a milk feed (either breast or bottle) you can begin to introduce some bland, mashed food, in small amounts.

At the start of the feed, try introducing one new food such as a vegetable puree, baby cereals, or fruit puree. One new food or drink at a time should be introduced, just in case it causes an upset in the baby, and to identify possible allergy.

Finger foods should be introduced at around six months, as babies like to hold their food. Items such as bread or toast, peeled slices of fruit or vegetables, small sandwiches, or slices of cheese are popular. Hard foods that cannot be softened in the mouth, such as hard candies or sweets, should be avoided to reduce risk of aspiration.

Parents should be reminded of the importance of supervising their child at all times, as babies can choke on food, and also to check that food is cool before placing it in front of the child, in order to prevent scalds.

17 Your primary assessment of any child with a history or recurrent/chronic otitis media with effusion is their speech and language development. These children are at a higher risk of a conductive hearing loss, due to the presence of persistent middle ear effusion. This effusion can be mild to severe in nature, being confirmed by an audiogram and tympanogram. These children may present with a very limited vocabulary and slurred speech, and often rely on visual aids and gesturing in communicating their needs. Audiograms should be done on all children with a speech and language delay, for chronic otitis media is often silent and goes undetected. The hearing loss usually resolves following surgical intervention (i.e. tympanotomy tubes). A repeat audiogram should be done following the surgical procedure to rule out the presence of any permanent/sensorineural hearing loss that may be present.

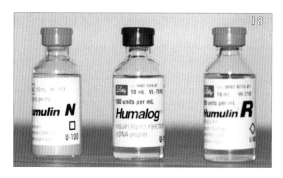

18 These insulins (**18**) are commonly prescribed for daily use to manage type 1 diabetes mellitus.
i. What are the major distinguishing characteristics of these insulins?
ii. How are these insulins administered in the daily self-care regimen?
iii. What self-care skill is taught in order for the patient/family to evaluate the effectiveness of the insulin dose?

19 This eight-month-old infant female with Down syndrome (**19**) is examined for an URI and conjunctivitis. Her mother reports that she has had repeated colds, with continuous nasal congestion for the past month, despite treatment with appropriate infant cold remedies as prescribed by her physician.
i. What common problems associated with Down syndrome should be ruled out for a child with this history?
ii. What signs and symptoms should be noted from this history?

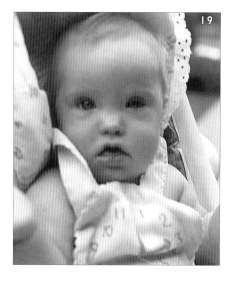

Insulin	Onset	Peak	Duration
Intermediate:			
NPH	1–2 hours	6–8 hours	12–15 hours
Lente	1–3 hours	6–12 hours	18–24 hours
Short:			
Regular	30 minutes	2–4 hours	4–8 hours
Lispro (Humalog)	10–15 minutes	0.5–1 hour	4 hours

18 i. These three types of insulin are unique in their action in relation to time: specifically, onset (time it takes to start working), peak (maximum effect time), and duration (how long it is biologically available to lower the blood glucose). Another distinguishing characteristic is their appearance. The intermediate-acting insulins, NPH or Lente (not pictured), are cloudy due to a preservative added to slow down their action. Short-acting Regular and Lispro (Humalog) insulins are clear. The time-course of action for these insulins is shown above.

Lispro (Humalog) insulin is especially useful because it more closely approximates the time–action of the endogenous insulin response of a normal pancreas at mealtime.
ii. Intermediate and short-acting insulins are typically mixed and given twice a day (split-mixed dose), before breakfast and before dinner, in order to provide 24-hour coverage with insulin. Each insulin peak occurs postprandially in order to utilize glucose absorbed at each meal. The extent of these peaks can be adjusted to meet an individual's requirement for insulin by raising or lowering the dose as needed.
iii. SBGM is the best method available at present, and permits a person with diabetes mellitus to determine their degree of control on a daily basis. Evaluating the efficacy of injected insulin is just one of the many reasons for SBGM. As children grow and develop over time, their need for insulin changes. Consistent, premeal, three to four times daily, SBGM can help alert parents and patients when a change of insulin dose is necessary.

19 i. Although approximately 40% of children with Down syndrome have significant heart lesions, including ventricular septal defects, transposition of great vessels, tetralogy of Fallot, hypoplastic left heart, and other severe structural heart lesions, significant cardiac findings may not be present in the first few days of life and go undetected until symptoms associated with cardiac failure emerge.
ii. This infant should be examined for signs of cardiac anomalies or respiratory symptoms underlying the continuous congestion reported by the parent. Heart and lung auscultation, signs of dyspnea, or changes in color should be observed if present.

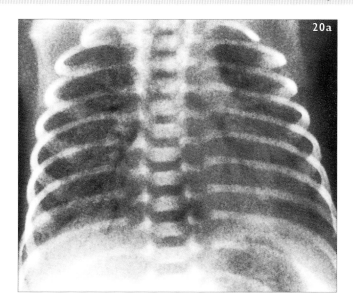

20 The child in this X-ray (**20a**) has BPD, the most frequently diagnosed chronic lung syndrome in preterm infants.
i. Summarize the clinical aspects of this disorder.
ii. Treatment of this chronic lung disease is primarily supportive and involves a complex array of medical therapies. The nurse must be knowledgeable about the principles of medical management. What does this medical management involve?
iii. What are the nursing considerations in managing the infant?

21 A child was diagnosed with acute lymphoblastic leukemia and has been started on a chemotherapy regimen consisting of prednisone, vincristine, and *Escherichia coli* asparaginase. Based on this photograph of a two-year-old child (**21**), list four methods to involve the child in accepting her medicine.

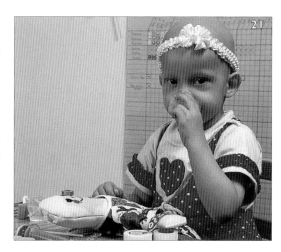

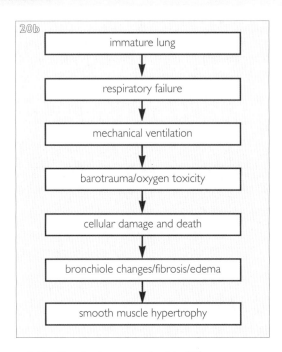

20b

immature lung

↓

respiratory failure

↓

mechanical ventilation

↓

barotrauma/oxygen toxicity

↓

cellular damage and death

↓

bronchiole changes/fibrosis/edema

↓

smooth muscle hypertrophy

20 i. The etiology of this disorder is summarized in **20b**.

ii. Medical management includes supplemental oxygen, bronchodilators, and anti-inflammatories.

iii. Ongoing nursing assessment is crucial in the care of this child. Respiratory assessment should include: signs and symptoms of distress, breath sounds, oxygenation assessment of the need for, and response to, treatment, and evaluation of the need for suctioning. Fluid status assessment should include: intake and output, daily weights, feeding tolerance, evaluation of electrolytes, and growth. Parent teaching and discharge planning should include developmental considerations.

21 Four methods are:

- Develop a sticker chart with all the medications listed for each day so that the child can mark with a sticker on the chart after each dose.
- Suggest that the child be given some reward such as one hour extra television time, a trip to the pet store, at the end of a specified time for successfully taking his/her medications (e.g. a week or a month).
- Allow the child to role-play, giving his/her doll or toy animal 'medications' first.
- Give the child choices with how or when to take medications (e.g. before or after dinner, with a syringe or a spoon).

22 A group of parents with school-age children ask for health and safety-related advice regarding athletic and physical activity plans for a summer camp.
i. At what age do gender-related physical features become significant in inter-sex athletic participation?
ii. Should male–female competition be discouraged at any particular age related to physical development and safety?

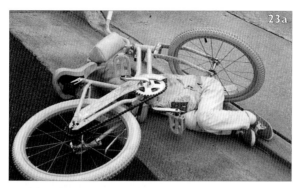

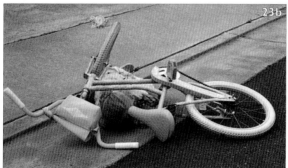

23 With no eye witnesses for this accident (**23a, b**), this child is found on the side of a quiet street. She is not responding to verbal calls and appears to be breathing, but is unconscious and not moving any extremities. There is no evidence of hemorrhage from the parts of her body that are visible.
i. Given her position and no explanation for how she may have fallen, what physical evidence can be assumed from what is visible?
ii. What are the first actions to be taken at the scene?
iii. What priorities must be set before removing the bicycle or turning the child over?
iv. What assessments can be made without equipment for possible head trauma?

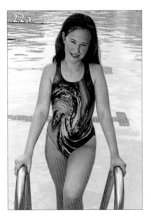
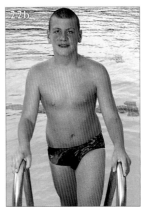

22 i. Before the age of 10, differences in physique and physical capabilities of males and females are difficult to differentiate. As children enter adolescence, the musculoskeletal framework of the male becomes greater in both relative and absolute terms. The children in **22a, b** are of same-age, prepubescent swimmers who are already showing signs of musculoskeletal changes. Males develop greater strength and power, and the farther along into puberty, the greater these differences become. Differential rates of pubertal progression cause extreme mismatches, even between males of the same age. The extent of such mismatches is far greater when pubescent males compete with pubescent females, particularly in sports where size, strength, and power are beneficial.

ii. In general, in relation to safety concerns for all at the summer camp, male–female competition and/or teams comprised of both males and females should be discontinued no later than the onset of pubertal progression.

23 i. Somehow, the child's body has become entangled under the bicycle, so one might assume that this has resulted from a fall. She has no helmet and she is unresponsive, therefore, one must suspect the possibility of head, neck, or back trauma, especially since she is not moving her extremities spontaneously.

ii. The first action is assessment of respiration and pulse. Since she is visibly breathing, the priority is to check the quality of her pulse by reaching in to an extremity.

iii. It is essential to keep her back and neck as immobilized as possible, turning her body as a unit only as necessary, and moving the bicycle off her body in order to continue assessing her respiratory status and possible sources of bleeding or injuries.

iv. The possibility of head trauma can be assessed better once she is supine and examined. Observing for physical evidence of head injury is the first line of assessment. Until medical help arrives, her level of consciousness should be checked frequently by calling out to her, stimulating her by touch, and checking her pupils for reactivity to light. Since she is breathing and a pulse can be palpated, the most important action is to keep her neck and body straight and in alignment.

24 An 18-month-old female comes to her mother from playing in another room. She is making incomprehensible noises, cannot close her mouth, and is drooling. Her mother sees a shiny object in the back of her mouth. She calls the emergency service. The ambulance arrives and transports her to the Emergency Department.

i. What does your assessment entail?

ii. What is the acceptable approach to the child with a partial airway obstruction from a foreign body?

iii. In addition to a portable lateral neck X-ray (**24**), what interventions should you prepare the patient and family for?

iv. What information should be included in your discharge teaching?

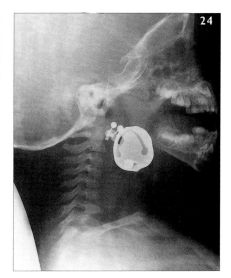

Medications	Vital signs
Prednisone 10 mg/day	Temperature 37°C (98.6°F)
Cyclosporin 250 mg/day	Pulse 76/min
Azathioprine (Imuran) 250 mg/day	BP 124/98 mmHg (16.5/13.1 kPa)
Laboratory values	*Weight*
Creatinine 97 μmol/l (1.1 mg/dl)	50 kg (110 lb)
Urea 2.2 mmol/l (BUN 13.0 mg/dl)	

25 A 14-year-old female presents at the renal clinic one year after renal transplant with complaint of recurrent headache. While the patient has received a renal transplant from her mother, she has never had her native kidneys removed. The adolescent denies any history of headaches before transplant. The patient and her mother state that the anti-rejection medication regimen has been strictly followed. The patient's blood pressure has been averaging 120/70 mmHg (16.0/9.3 kPa). The patient's laboratory data are shown above.

i. Considering her renal history, what significance could the presence of a headache have for this adolescent? What other factors could be contributing to the headache?

ii. When assessing hypertension in individuals after renal transplant, what part of the medical history is important to obtain?

iii. What other factors besides rejection might account for the increase in blood pressure?

24 i. Your assessment begins with an observation for airway patency to ensure oxygenation will be optimal. If the airway is not patent, open it by performing the BLS maneuvers of head-tilt chin-lift, or jaw thrust action, begin oxygen therapy, and proceed with your assessment of breathing and circulation status.

ii. If you suspect a foreign body aspiration or obstruction, encourage the child to cough forcefully. A blind finger sweep of the mouth of an infant or child should be avoided to prevent pushing the object further back and resulting in complete airway obstruction. Allow the child to sit, comforted by a parent, in an upright position until the foreign body can be extracted in a controlled manner in the presence of supportive personnel, such as an anesthesiologist and respiratory therapist.

iii. You should prepare the child and family for a portable lateral neck and chest X-ray to assist with defining the location and structure of the object causing obstruction. Preparation should also include emergency preoperative teaching for a patient undergoing a bronchoscopy or esophagoscopy. The brief postoperative recovery period should also be discussed.

iv. Discharge teaching regarding postoperative care includes observation of the child for respiratory distress, temperature, poor oral intake or swallowing difficulties, and anxiety secondary to the emergent event. Injury prevention information regarding small objects and food materials should also be shared with the family. Small objects less than 3 cm (1 in) should not be within the reach of a child less than three years old.

25 i. A transplant recipient's complaint of headaches, as with any individual's complaint of headache, needs to be assessed thoroughly to identify the cause of the pain. The cause of elevated blood pressure must also be assessed, as hypertension alone can cause individuals to have headaches. While a headache or an elevated blood pressure could be a sign of transplant rejection, there are other possible explanations for the complaint of headache and hypertension, such as stress.

ii. Initially, it is important to obtain a complete medical/social history of the individual as appropriate for any female adolescent. Then, it is important to examine the renal medical history, including the type and cause of their primary renal disease.

iii. The blood pressure could increase due to a wide range of factors, such as damage or return of disease in the transplanted kidney, structural changes or problems, side-effects of immunosuppression, malignant neoplasms, and the presence of the native kidneys.

26 A two-year-old female has only recently begun to walk (16 months) and demonstrates questionable motor coordination, mild ataxia, and poor muscle tone.
i. A comfortable position for her is shown (26). What is this position called, and why is it comfortable for her?
ii. Why should she or should she not be encouraged to be positioned in this manner?

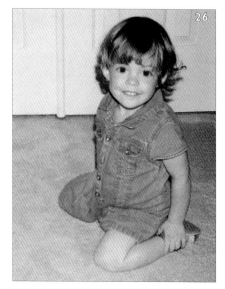

27 A previously healthy nine-month-old infant is brought to the Emergency Department twice within three days, with a history of irritability, poor feeding, and listlessness. The initial visit described an infant that was irritable; however, the physical examination was within normal limits. The infant was diagnosed with a 'virus' and was discharged with instructions to follow-up with the pediatrician. Three days later, notes from a second Emergency Department visit documented an infant who was listless, fed poorly from the bottle, and was extremely irritable. The remainder of the examination was within normal limits. There was no evidence of external trauma to the infant. The parents of the infant are 20 years old, not married, and both describe 'tension' with the grandparents. The mother is employed and provides the insurance coverage. The father is out of work. The parents reside in an apartment for 'low-income' families. Both parents are attentive to the child and display appropriate concern with the child's illness. They deny any history of trauma. A possible diagnosis of SBS has been made.
i. While taking the 'history' from the family and during the examination of the infant, what information may indicate that this family is at risk for child abuse (SBS)? What characteristics does this family reflect?
ii. When the nurse is obtaining the history from the family, what would be appropriate assessment strategies?

26 i. Sitting in the W position is comfortable for a child with poor coordination or muscle tone because it provides a feeling of stability from which to interact with toys. **ii.** Hip subluxation or dislocation may occur in infants or toddlers with markedly increased adductor tone at the hips. Prolonged sitting in the W position, especially in a child with tonal abnormalities, may predispose to this condition.

27 i. This family reflects several of the behaviors shown in the three columns of the table below, including parental immaturity, financial stress, unemployment, lack of family support, and a difficult temperament in the infant.

Characteristics of the parents	Other factors	Characteristics of the child
Unrealistic expectations of the child	Substance abuse	Physical anomalies
Poor nurturing or abuse during childhood	Financial difficulties	Physical/developmental delay
Low self-esteem or depression	Unemployment	Difficult temperament
Parental immaturity	Divorce	Reminds parents of someone 'negatively'
Inadequate knowledge of normal development	Relationship difficulties	Does not meet parent's expectations
Substance abuse	Lack of family support	
Financial stress or social isolation	Difficulty controlling impulses	

ii. (1) Inquiries must be made about the infant's past medical history, allergies, medications, babysitters, and regular caregivers. (2) The parents and caregivers should be interviewed separately and should be asked about the 'details' that brought the infant to the Emergency Department and if an injury occurred; any inconsistencies between parties concerning the description of the injury should be noted as well as any explanations that are inconsistent with the clinical picture. (3) A meticulous examination of the infant, including less obvious bruising or other injuries that may have been missed (small oval bruises on the infant's upper arms may be thumbprint marks). (4) Parent/caregivers should be questioned about the temperament of the infant, as infants who are described as 'colicky', 'hard to settle', and 'inconsolable crying', are at a higher risk for SBS. Ask the parents/caregivers how they are dealing with the infant, e.g. are they getting enough sleep, and do they have family who can help care for the child? This will help to identify such conditions as lack of sleep and frustration.

28 This six-month-old female premature baby (28) has a tracheostomy tube. How is it best to suction a tracheostomy tube in an infant?

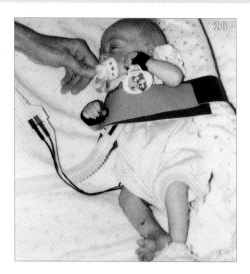

Response to exercise challenge

Cycle time	FEV$_1$ (l)	Change (%)
Baseline	4.0	
0 min postexercise	3.8	5
10 min postexercise	3.4	15
15 min postexercise	3.0	25
20 min postbronchodilator	3.7	23

29 A 15-year-old, white female who plays on the high school soccer team reports to the pulmonary clinic with the following complaints: two-week occurrence of shortness of breath while running up and down the field, accompanied by chest tightness and a cough. She has a normal chest examination and office spirometry (see table). However, the physician suspects EIA and orders an exercise challenge. The results are positive and the patient is prescribed a bronchodilator to be used 15–20 minutes before exercise and after exercise if needed. If the patient is still having problems during the soccer game, she is told to call for the addition of a long-acting bronchodilator.
i. Why were the lung examination and spirometry normal?
ii. What should you tell the teenager about what will happen during an exercise challenge? How does an exercise challenge confirm the diagnosis of asthma? Looking at the patient's chart, did the teenager demonstrate a response to exercise?
iii. What rationale can you give the patient for how a bronchodilator medication prevents or decreases EIA?

28 Vacuum pressure should range between 80–100 mmHg (10.6–13.3 kPa). The suction catheter should have a diameter of no larger than one-half the diameter of the tracheostomy tube in order to prevent obliteration of the tracheostomy tube during suctioning. The suction catheter should not be advanced until resistance is met, as this has been shown to cause trauma to the tracheobronchial wall. The suction catheter should be inserted to a premeasured depth ≤0.5 cm (≤0.2 in) beyond the tip of the tracheostomy tube. A small amount of sterile isotonic saline may be injected into the tracheostomy tube to help loosen secretions for ease of aspiration. Hyperoxygenation with oxygen before and after each aspiration should be performed to prevent hypoxia. The infant should be allowed to rest for 30–60 seconds after each aspiration.

29 i. A person with a chronic disease such as asthma will not always demonstrate symptoms, especially if the asthma is not active. Therefore, when a patient presents with shortness of breath, cough, and tightness in the chest, but both the spirometry and chest examination are normal, a diagnosis of asthma can not be ruled out. It may be necessary to recreate the precipitating event in order to demonstrate the change in lung function and reproduce the symptoms.
ii. The exercise challenge is used to determine the degree of airway irritability and to measure the response to treatment. There are several ways to perform an exercise challenge. During the challenge the teenager must increase her heart rate by 80% for 4–6 minutes. She will run in place for several minutes, and then undergo a set of pulmonary function tests to see if there is a change in FEV_1. A more sophisticated test uses a stationary bicycle or treadmill, so that the time and degree of activity are regulated. These tests can provoke a mild form of asthma and chest tightness in a teenager with asthma that can be reversed in 10–20 minutes with bronchodilator therapy. This was demonstrated in this patient with at least a 15% drop in FEV_1 and a reversal of at least 15%.
iii. Short-acting bronchodilators relax airway smooth muscles and increase airflow. They are the drugs of choice in preventing EIA and treating acute asthma symptoms and exacerbations. Because the medications take from 5–30 minutes to work, they are taken 20–30 minutes before exercise. Their effect may last 2–3 hours. A 10- to 15-minute warm up period before exercise will also help. EIA should be anticipated in all asthma patients and addressed accordingly. It can be caused by loss of heat and moisture in the lungs during exercise due to hyperventilation. It usually starts during or shortly after the activity and lasts for 15–20 minutes.

30 This normal eight-year-old female (30a) has had some difficulties in school, as reported by her teacher, since the beginning of spring. She has had difficulty completing her work and is demonstrating several irritating behaviors. Her eyes are itchy and red from rubbing, with darker, swollen marks underneath.

i. What signs and behaviors are indicative of allergic rhinitis and how do they evolve?

ii. What possible sequelae might result from these long-term behaviors?

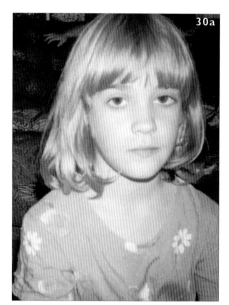

	Breakfast	Lunch	Dinner	Bedtime
Monday	6.10 (114)	12.0 (223)	6.42 (119)	7.75 (144)
Tuesday	6.41 (119)	12.3 (229)	7.10 (132)	7.30 (136)
Wednesday	5.29 (98)	10.5 (195)	6.39 (118)	7.75 (144)
Thursday	6.42 (119)	11.0 (205)	5.80 (108)	7.50 (140)
Friday	5.25 (98)	12.8 (230)		

31 A 10-year-old male with a four-year history of type 1 diabetes mellitus who weighs 35 kg (77 lb) has the above blood glucose pattern (concentrations in mmol/l [mg/dl]). His current insulin dose is 8 units of NPH plus 3 units of Regular insulin before breakfast, and 3 units of NPH plus 2 units of Regular insulin before dinner.

i. Is this insulin dose appropriate for this child's needs?

ii. What needs to be done in order to correct the present pattern?

iii. Would decreasing the morning food intake have the same effect on the blood glucose pattern?

iv. What other questions need to be asked in order to analyze fully the blood glucose pattern?

30 i. Allergic 'shiners' (discoloration around the eyes) (**30a**), the 'allergic salute' (**30b**), and facial twitching or grimacing are very common signs and behaviors in children with allergic rhinitis. The fingers and palms rubbed over the nose are accompanied by sniffling. The origin of these irritating behaviors is nasal itching but, once established, the mannerism may persist beyond successful treatment of the rhinitis.

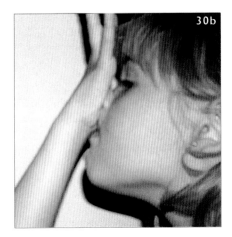

ii. In the long term, a permanent transverse nasal crease may result.

31 i. No. The average dose of insulin for children is around 0.8–1 unit/kg/day. This child is on 16 units per day, or 0.46 unit/kg/day.

ii. In order to correct the pattern of hyperglycemia noted at lunch time, more regular insulin needs to be administered in the morning. A 10–15% increase in the morning regular insulin will prevent hyperglycemia by lunch time.

iii. Perhaps, but withholding food is generally not a good idea. Children need enough calories and the right amount of insulin for growth. If a child with diabetes mellitus shows an appropriate rate of growth over time for age, the blood glucose level should be controlled with insulin, not food. As long as the meal pattern is consistent and reasonable, no change should be made in diet at this time.

iv. Prior to changing the insulin dose, all other contributing factors that need modification should be assessed, such as recent infection, change in schedule, dramatic drop in activity level, and/or stress.

32 When a child has a tracheostomy, the upper airway is bypassed.
i. What important functions of the upper airway must we now provide for the child?

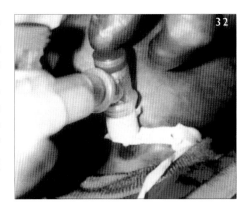

During January while her brother has a cold, this infant (32) begins demonstrating rhinorrhea, congestion, dyspnea, cough, wheezing, fever, lethargy, and poor feeding.
ii. What is the likely etiology and treatment?

33 This 16-year-old female (33) is admitted to the hospital for cystic fibrosis, severe chronic obstructive pulmonary disease, and lung transplant evaluation. She recently began sleeping up to 12 hours per night, awakening often with cough, plus two naps during the day. She experiences increasing dyspnea with walking stairs and distances greater than one block. She has active inspiratory and expiratory wheezing and a less productive cough. Medications include furosemide 60 mg daily, prednisone 60 mg daily, KCl 30 mEq daily, and tobramycin 120 mg t.i.d. via aerosol.

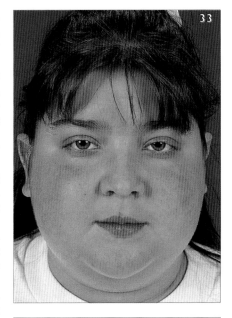

i. What major developmental issues would the patient be concerned about? What nursing strategies can be utilized to support her in dealing with these issues?
ii. What is the rationale for her medication regimen? Which side-effects are most significant to her?

Her most recent laboratory results are shown.
iii. How can these be interpreted?

Na 136 mmol/l (mEq/l) (135–145*)
K 3.2 mmol/l (mEq/l) (3.5–5.5*)
Cl 96 mmol/l (mEq/l) (98–108*)
CO_2 26 mmol/l (mEq/l) (23–30*)
HGB A_{1c} 6.1%
*Normal range

32 & 33: Answers

32 i. When an infant with a tracheostomy is cared for, the airway must be provided with warmth, humidity, and filtration, which would normally be done by the upper airway.
ii. RSV is a common seasonal lower respiratory illness in at-risk infants, especially those with BPD, who are preterm, or who have congenital heart disease. Treatment is supportive and may include oxygen, fluid therapy, and bronchodilators. Nursing care includes assessment and structuring intervention for maximal rest and minimal energy expenditure. Parents should be counseled that this illness is best prevented through good hand washing and avoiding contact with at-risk populations such as day-care centers in the winter months, if the child would be placed in peril by a RSV infection.

33 i. The teenager with cystic fibrosis has concerns about socialization with peers and maintaining contact with fellow students during periods of hospitalization. Body image concerns are equally important. Allow the teenager to socialize with classmates as much as possible by planning hospitalizations for cystic fibrosis exacerbations around school vacation times or utilize home intravenous antibiotics when possible.
ii. Respiratory failure and cor pulmonale develop as cystic fibrosis progresses. Steroid therapy may prevent pulmonary fibrosis. However, it can cause moon facies, growth retardation, hypertension, and glucose abnormalities. Furosemide (Lasix) is utilized in overt heart failure, most often in cystic fibrosis hypertrophy of the right ventricle. It can alter fluid and electrolyte balance. KCl replaces potassium lost as a result of furosemide and chronic steroid therapy. Headaches and cardiac irregularities are common side-effects. Tobramycin is an aerosolized antibiotic with the primary side-effects of high-frequency deafness.
iii. Diuretic and chronic steroid therapy are causing fluid and electrolyte imbalance. Hypokalemia and hypochloremia can be corrected by altering the doses of furosemide and oral potassium. Hemoglobin A_{1c} indicates potential glucose abnormalities.

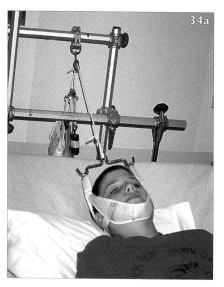

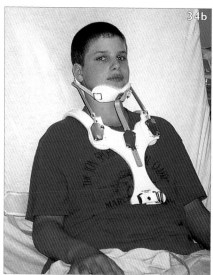

34 An 11-year-old male sustained a cervical 6 spinous process fracture and perched facet C6–C7 after being struck by a motor vehicle while riding his bike. He was placed into a cervical head halter (34a) for reduction. He remained in this traction for four days and was then placed in a somi brace (34b) for discharge home.

i. What type of traction is a cervical head halter?

ii. What must be included in the nurse's assessment of a patient in a cervical head halter?

iii. What discharge teaching related to skin care must be done with a patient being discharged to home in a brace?

35 This child (35), who is ventilator-dependent and has a tracheostomy, is being prepared for an outing. In addition to being adequately supervised by a trained caregiver, the child should be in a portable environment that has been prepared for unexpected emergencies.

i. What resources and equipment must be included with the ventilated child?

ii. What emergencies should be planned for?

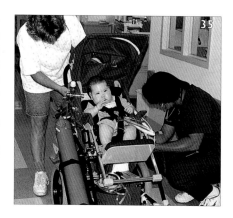

34 i. A cervical head halter is a form of skin traction which is used to treat mild cervical trauma. A cervical head halter applies pulling g force directly to the patient's skin and soft tissue and indirectly to the skeletal structures, thereby immobilizing the neck yet helping to relieve muscle spasms and compression of the nerves. Due to the risk of skin irritation, skin traction is used intermittently with lighter weights and for a shorter duration than skeletal traction.

ii. Pressure on the skin is the major concern with any form of skin traction. The chin, ears, mandibular joint, and occiput must be carefully assessed. The patient should also be assessed for jaw pain, which would indicate too much weight. Frequent neurologic checks should be done, including pupil size and reaction, level of consciousness, orientation to person, place and time, extremity strength, and hand grasps.

iii. Skin irritation and breakdown are common complications associated with bracing. These problems can be avoided with meticulous skin care. Patients should be instructed to assess and wash the skin under their brace twice a day. They should be taught to watch for pink or red areas that can progress to raw skin. After washing, rubbing alcohol should be applied to all areas covered by the brace to help toughen the skin. Special attention should be applied to bony areas such as the hips, shoulders, and ribs. Creams, powders, and lotions should not be used under the brace because they soften the skin and are difficult to clean from the brace. A smooth, unwrinkled, snug-fitting cotton T-shirt or cotton tube should be worn under the brace at all times to avoid direct skin and brace contact. These undergarments should be changed and laundered daily.

35 i. The child's stroller should have all of the oxygen and equipment necessary to sustain ventilation for the length of time the child will be away. In addition, there should be one extra same-size tracheostomy tube, one smaller tracheostomy tube, scissors, and ties. Suction tubing and saline should be easily available in the stroller and a suction unit should accompany the ventilator unit. An ambu bag with both a tracheostomy adaptor and mask should also be visible for emergencies.

ii. In addition to specific child complications anticipated and planned for such as the tracheostomy tube becoming plugged or dislodged, equipment malfunction should always be a possibility that the caregivers anticipate. While the ambu bag with oxygen support can provide some temporary ventilation, equipment malfunction should be prevented by good maintenance and testing prior to any outing.

36 What are the principles of caring for a gastrostomy stoma and the skin around it?

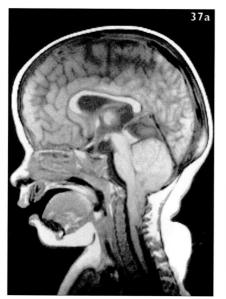
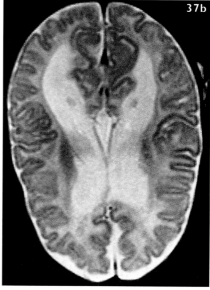

37 A full-term infant with an L4–L5 myelomeningocele was delivered by cesarean section. Closure of the back defect was performed at 12 hours of age.
i. What are two findings commonly seen in children with a myelomeningocele (37a, b)?
ii. What observations may indicate that the child is experiencing increased intracranial pressure and may require shunt placement due to hydrocephalus?
iii. What observations of this infant may indicate a symptomatic Chiari II malformation?
iv. What other assessments should the nurse make regarding the infant's sensory and motor function?

36 Keep the skin around the gastrostomy healthy. Assess the site routinely, at least during each feeding. Rinse and dry the area daily to keep it clean and dry. Use gauze, cotton tipped applicators, and/or a soft cloth to cleanse the skin and tube. Clean the underside of the ring and rotate the tube to prevent it from adhering to the stoma tract. Mild soap and warm water should be used. Gently remove encrustations from around and underneath the disc (36). Half-strength hydrogen peroxide may be recommended for signs of skin breakdown or drainage. Rinse with water to prevent the skin from drying out. Aseptic technique is essential to prevent bacterial infection. Report any redness, irritation, soreness, or unusual drainage.

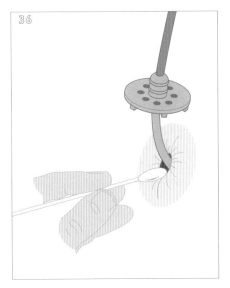

37 i. Enlarged ventricles (37a) indicate hydrocephalus which occurs in 80–90% of children with myelomeningocele. A Chiari II malformation (37b) in which portions of the hindbrain extend into the spinal canal occurs in more than 80% of children with myelomeningocele.

ii. There are several signs/symptoms that may indicate a child is experiencing increased intracranial pressure due to hydrocephalus. These are:

- Increased head circumference.
- Bulging fontanelles.
- Prominent scalp veins or forehead.
- Irritability.
- Vomiting.

iii. Signs of a symptomatic Chiari II malformation may include:

- Inspiratory stridor.
- Difficulty in swallowing.
- Sustained arching of the head.
- A weak cry.

iv. The nurse should assess the infant for signs of a neurogenic bladder and/or neurogenic bowel. An infant with a neurogenic bladder tends to drip urine on a continual basis, or has a distended bladder. The infant should also be monitored for constipation as this may be the presenting sign of a neurogenic bowel. Frequent evaluation of the skin for injury due to pressure or other trauma should be performed as skin innervated from affected nerves will usually have altered sensation and function. The evaluation of the skin should include the diaper area which should be observed for rashes or skin breakdown due to contact with urine and/or stool.

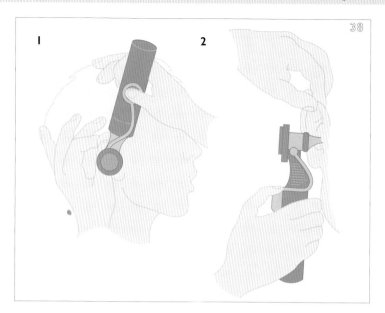

38 An unhappy and apprehensive three-year-old needs an otoscopic examination for history of fever, malaise, poor appetite, and complaint of ear pain. With some coaxing, he is willing to have his ear examined.
i. Which of the figures (38 (1), (2)) shows the best otoscope positioning that should be used and why?
ii. What other precautions might be taken for this procedure?

39 This nine-month-old female (39) is having great fun playing. Taking the four key areas of development, what milestones would you antici-pate a nine-month-old child to achieve with relation to:
i. Posture and large move-ment?
ii. Vision and fine movement?
iii. Hearing and speech?
iv. Social behavior and play?

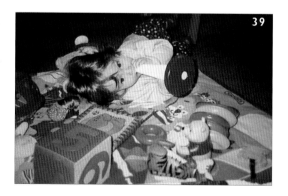

38 i. Positioning the otoscope with both hands (38 (1)) will enhance visualization and minimize the chance that head movement will result in trauma to the ear canal, particularly if the behavior of the child is unknown and could erupt at any moment. When the child is cooperative, a finger touching the cheek is sufficient to stabilize the tip inside the ear (38 (2)).
ii. If the child's behavior is unpredictable and mother is present, she could be encouraged to hold the child on her lap and stabilize the child's head with a gentle, firm arm, while holding the child's hands within her hand.

39 i. Nine-month-old children are able to sit alone for 10–15 minutes on the floor, will lean forward to pick up a toy without losing balance, and may turn their body to look sideways or pick an item up from the floor. When sitting in the pram, cot, or bath, they will demonstrate very active movements of body and all limbs. Children make a great deal of effort to crawl, and may be successful. If they are unable to crawl, they tend to roll or squirm on the floor to facilitate mobility.

Nine-month-old children may also try to pull themselves up into a standing position, but are unable to lower themselves and thus fall backwards to a sitting position. If held in a standing position, infants have a tendency to make purposeful stepping movements.
ii. Visually, infants are very attentive to everyone and everything in their environment. They stretch out to reach toys, with one hand dominating, and like to pass things from hand to hand. They drop toys but cannot place them down in a voluntary fashion. They look in the right direction for falling or fallen toys, particularly those that have fallen from a cot/pram (crib). They are beginning to develop fine movements between finger and thumb, and can pick up a small sweet with a pincer movement.
iii. Infants are very attentive to normal everyday sounds with particular emphasis on voices. They make vocal noises as a way to communicate friendliness or anger/frustration, with babbling noises or shouting. Babbling can be quite tuneful, such as dad-dad, mam-mam, adada, or agaga.
iv. Infants will hold their bottle or cup when feeding, try to grasp a spoon when feeding, and will hold, bite, and chew a biscuit. If approached by unfamiliar people, they will cling to the familiar person and require reassurance before accepting their advances. They will cling to the known adult and hide their face. All objects are taken to the mouth. They like to play peek-a-boo, imitate hand clapping, and wave toys around to make a noise, e.g. bells/rattles.

40 This toddler returned to day care following a two-day absence for treatment of pediculosis diagnosed by the pediatrician. The parent reports that she washed the child's head with the prescribed anti-lice shampoo.
i. What does the parent need to check for prior to sending the child back to day care?
ii. What do the nits (eggs) observed on the child's hair shafts (**40**) indicate? What must be done?

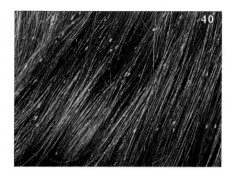

Time	01:00	02:00	03:00
Plasma acetone	Large		Moderate
Blood glucose (fasting) (3.8–5.9 mmol/l [70–110 mg/dl])*	29.5 (550)	22.0 (410)	11.3 (210)
K (3.5–5.5 mmol/l [mEq/l])*	5.8		3.5
CO_2 (23–30 mmol/l [mEq/l])*	9		14
Na (135–145 mmol/l [mEq/l])*	134		149
Cl (98–108 mmol/l [mEq/l])*	109		108
pH (7.35–7.45)*	7.10		7.21
Urea (1.2–3.0 mmol/l [BUN 7.0–18.0 mg/dl])*	3.3 (20.0)		3.0 (18.0)
*Normal range			

41 A 14-year-old male with a six-year history of type 1 diabetes mellitus came into the Emergency Department in DKA. He also had a two-day history of nausea and vomiting, and high concentrations of ketones in the urine. Your assessment reveals that this adolescent has been giving his own injections since onset. Recently, his parents announced they were getting a divorce and his father moved out of the house. The initial blood work is shown above.
  On admission to the Emergency Department, the youth was given an intravenous fluid bolus of 0.9% normal saline over one hour. An insulin drip was started at 0.1 units/kg/hr along with 0.45% normal saline with 10 mmol/l (mEq/l) KCl and 10 mmol/l (mEq/l) K-phosphate at maintenance/replacement rate. The patient is no longer vomiting, but remains nauseated and NPO.
i. In light of the blood glucose at this time, what change needs to be made in the intravenous fluid administration?
ii. Blood was sent for a glycosylated hemoglobin A_{1c} test and was 15% (normal 3–6%). What does this mean? How might this result suggest a possible reason for his DKA?
iii. What may be a necessary intervention for this adolescent and his parents to prevent further deterioration of metabolic control?

40 i. It is not sufficient merely to shampoo a child with pediculosis because the solutions may not kill the head lice and do not remove the nits already left on the shafts of hair. The parent needs to inspect for nits that are visible and be sure that they are removed before the child is allowed to be in group care.
ii. The nits indicate that the lice had sufficient time to leave eggs and the special nit comb should be used to comb the hair and remove the eggs.

41 i. When plasma glucose decreases to 13.4 mmol/l (250 mg/dl), the intravenous fluids need to be changed to a fluid with glucose. Since the patient is still acidotic (pH 7.21) he still needs insulin to allow for the utilization of glucose as an energy substrate. The process of ketone production must be stopped. It is a mistake to lower the rate of the insulin drip at this time. Intravenous fluids with dextrose solutions (D5 to D10% glucose) will provide a ready supply of glucose for the insulin to work on and prevent hypoglycemia. Prevention of hypoglycemia is essential because of the accompanying glucose-raising effect of counter-regulatory hormones.
ii. This test measures hemoglobin from red blood cells to which glucose has become irreversibly attached by nonenzymatic means. This attachment of glucose (glycosylation) occurs slowly; therefore, the amount of glycosylation is proportional to the average level of blood sugar over the past two to three months (or the lifespan of the red blood cell). The glycosylated hemoglobin test measures the overall success of the diabetes mellitus management program. In fact, it represents glucose conditions over a very extended period of time. A glycosylated hemoglobin of <8% means that the average blood glucose has remained in the normal range over the past two to three months and the diabetes mellitus is under excellent control. When the hemoglobin A_{1c} is >11%, it means the patient is probably missing some insulin injections. Omitting insulin is a common cause of DKA in adolescence.
iii. This adolescent and his family will need an assessment to evaluate the degree to which the changes occurring in the family structure impact on his ability to manage his illness. Individual, group, or family therapy may help him cope with his adolescence, a chronic illness, and life in general.

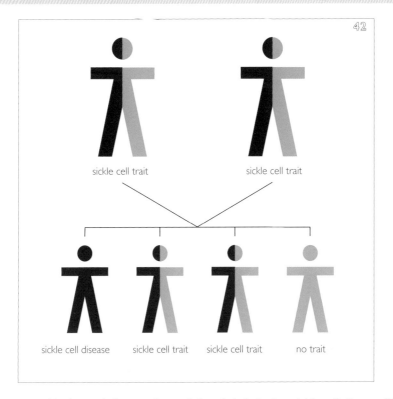

42 A young, black couple has just learned that their baby has sickle cell disease. They wonder how this could happen. Neither parent knows of any relative having been told that they are carriers of the disease and no one has had sickle cell disease. They are immediately sent to the genetic counselor to understand their likelihood of having other children with the disease.

Using the chart (**42**), what can this anxious couple be told about the chances of having a second child with sickle cell disease?

43 A six-month-old infant with a history of perinatal anoxia (APGARs 3 and 6 at one and five minutes) is assessed for neurologic sequelae from birth history. Neurologic reflexes are tested and compared with earlier developmental examinations.
i. What are some of the primitive reflexes called, and how would they be checked?
ii. Which reflexes should be present in a normal six-month-old, and when should they disappear?

42 This unpleasant news comes as a result of both parents being carriers of sickle cell trait and not knowing. When each parent is a carrier of sickle cell trait, there are three possible outcomes with each pregnancy: 50% chance of having a child with sickle cell trait who may in the future parent a child with sickle cell disease; 25% chance of having a child with sickle cell disease; 25% chance of having a child without trait or disease.

43 i. The reflexes shown are: (**43 (1)**) parachute, checked by tilting the child's head and torso towards the ground causing the infant to spread arms and legs out; (**43 (2)**) Perez reflex, checked by applying finger pressure along the spine of a horizontally suspended infant in a caudal–cephalad direction causing flexion of the arms and legs, elevation of the head and a sudden cry; (**43 (3)**) Galant reflex, checked by stroking the skin in the lumbar para-vertebral area, causing arching of the trunk towards the stimulated side.

ii. The intact six-month-old should still demonstrate a Perez reflex, which disappears between 4–6 months, should have lost the Galant reflex, which disappears between 2–3 months, and will not yet demonstrate the parachute reflex, which generally does not appear until 7–9 months and persists.

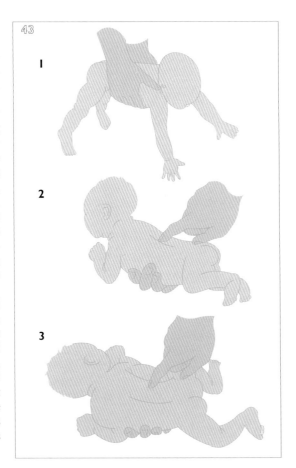

44 A 16-year-old male was diving off a bridge into the ocean. The tide had changed and he struck the frontoparietal area of his head on the ocean floor. He walked out of the water complaining of discomfort over his upper cervical vertebrae and he felt weakness in his arms and legs with an intermittent tingling sensation through his extremities to his digits. His friends put him in the car and drove to the local hospital.
i. What would be the first intervention upon arrival at the hospital?
ii. What should the nurse anticipate and prepare the patient for in terms of evaluation and procedures?
iii. Which immobilization options will be considered for the patient with cervical spinal cord or column injury?
iv. What teaching should be done with the patient and family if a Halo brace jacket (44a) is applied?

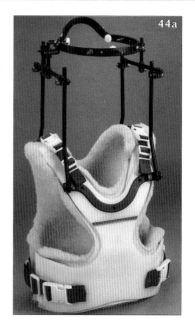

45 A five-year-old male has acute lymphoblastic leukemia. He requires frequent spinal taps as part of his treatment to monitor the central nervous system for spread of his leukemia (45). He is afraid that the spinal taps will be painful and worries that he will move and 'they will have to poke me again'. The mother asks you how to assist and comfort her son through these procedures. What suggestions would you give the mother?

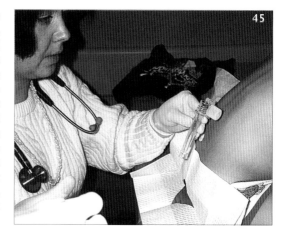

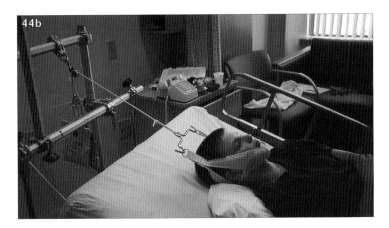

44 i. Upon arrival at the hospital and after rapid assessment of airway, breathing and circulation are complete, the patient should be placed in a hard (extrication) cervical collar with his head in neutral position. He should then be placed on a long backboard with head blocks in place (44b) and instructed to remain supine until directed otherwise.

ii. The patient should be prepared for a complete secondary survey with a thorough neurologic and musculoskeletal assessment. The cranial nerves will be tested, as well as the spinal reflexes. An intravenous line will be started with a high-dose methylpredniso-lone drip. X-rays will include lateral, anterior–posterior and odontoid views of the cervical spine. A cervical CT and MRI will be carried out.

iii. Commonly prescribed procedures for treatment of cervical spine injuries include immobilization and surgery. Immobilization can be with orthotics, such as hard cervical collars or skeletal or skin traction. Skeletal traction may be applied to the patient confined to bed. Halo skeletal traction may be used in bed, in a wheelchair, or with a (vest) jacket apparatus for an ambulatory patient. Skin traction with a chin halter and straps can be used intermittently for more stable injuries. The goals of cervical orthotics are support and immobilization.

iv. If a Halo brace (vest) jacket is applied, teaching for the patient and family includes personal hygiene, activity restriction, injury prevention, such as balance education and automobile travel safety, and skin care for the pins and under the vest. Signs that need to be reported to the physician immediately include pin loosening, pain, or pin site drainage. Surgery (fusions, laminectomies, or decompressions) may be required to stabilize the cervical injury prior to the orthotic application.

45 Suggestions are:

- Create a calm atmosphere with his favorite music (headphones).
- Work on his breathing to relax him (slow deep breaths).
- Distract him with bubbles, kaleidoscope, and/or picture books.
- Use imagery – 'let's talk about your birthday party ... pet ... or favorite room at home'.

46 A nine-year-old female was born with exstrophy of the bladder and has undergone, over her nine years, a series of reconstructive surgeries. These included an operation to close the bladder, lengthen the bladder neck, with subsequent repairs, and reconstruction of a large bladder reservoir to augment the bladder. Because the augmented bladder was unable to contract normally, it needs catheterization in order for it to be emptied. A special channel from the bladder to the umbilicus was created that does not leak and is easy to catheterize (**46**).

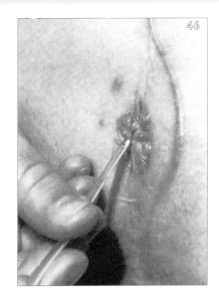

i. What nursing care and patient education is essential to the long-term success of the procedure?
ii. What care is necessary for the girl in self-catheterizing to minimize infection?

47 This two-year-old female (**47**) is brought to the Emergency Department by her mother. The girl has bruises on the side of her face extending to the outer ear. The mother says that the child walked into a door.

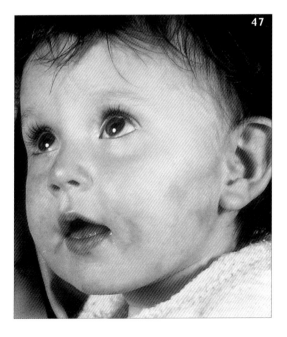

i. What would be the immediate nursing intervention/observations for the nurse to make?
ii. What could facial bruising indicate in this child?
iii. What other signs could indicate long-term abuse in a two-year-old child?

46 i. Once the stoma healed and the suprapubic catheter was removed, the girl needed to be taught to catheterize herself. She needed to trust that it would not be painful and to do whatever manipulation was needed to pass the catheter into the bladder. She needed to learn to flush the catheter with a concentrated solution of normal saline whenever it became plugged with mucus. Her family needed to learn how to trouble-shoot and help support her in her self-care.
ii. Careful handwashing and a nightly antibiotic help minimize infection.

47 i. This child has sustained a head injury, at this stage the cause is unknown. Standard head injury observations should be commenced, i.e. level of consciousness, blood pressure, pupil reaction, active/passive state of child. The child should also be examined for any other injury. Gentle 'open' questioning of the child may yield an explanation.
ii. Bruising, such as in this child, is very unlikely to be caused by walking into a door, the mother's explanation. Therefore, physical abuse should be suspected.

Child protection procedures must be followed. In the UK, child protection guidance has been drawn up by local Area Child Protection Committees and specifies each agency's role in protecting the child. In the USA, child protection laws mandate reporting.

The consultant pediatrician and designated doctor must be notified and it is his/her duty to speak to the parent(s). A full exploration of the facts is essential and the medical staff must inform parents of the need to evaluate further the situation in partnership with the Social Services Department and Police.

Health Visitors and School Nurses hold valuable records about each child; there-fore, liaison with the relevant individual is essential to obtain a retrospective history of the child's health.

The importance of record-keeping cannot be overestimated, as records may be required for case conferences or court proceedings.
iii. Emergency departments keep records of attendance. This child may have a history of minor injuries or have attended other local Emergency Departments. The child's school should be contacted for information about attendance, behavior, and social skills, as well as educational ability.

Growth is an important indicator of the child's well-being. Small stature and failure to thrive can be a result of emotional abuse. Height measurements must be taken accurately over a period of several months to ascertain true height velocity. Children who are unhappy grow and develop slowly.

Domestic violence must also be considered. The child's bruises could be the result of a single episode of loss of temper, or be a part of a long-term violent relationship between parents which has escalated, involving the children.

The priority in all cases is the safety of the child. No single agency, or person, has the authority to make decisions. All decisions regarding protection of children should be made by the multidisciplinary team.

48 The child with Down syndrome is usually diagnosed at birth. Although the etiology is unclear, the cytogenetics are well known.
i. What are the genetic manifestations of Down syndrome, and which is the most common?
ii. What is the nurse's role in the early phase of diagnosis?

49 An 18-year-old female has been diagnosed with osteogenic sarcoma. She refuses to talk about receiving chemotherapy because she has no one to stay with her one-year-old and three-year-old children when she is in the hospital. You advise her that there are ways for her to receive some of her treatment at home (**49**). What two methods could you advise her about?

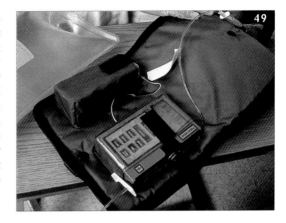

50 This 10-month-old infant (**50**) has a nasojejunal tube secondary to severe gastro-esophageal reflux resistant to antacids, prokinetics, thickened feeds, and positioning.
i. How do you measure for nasojejunal tube placement in an infant or toddler?
ii. What clinical data, other than an X-ray, suggest proper placement in the jejunum?

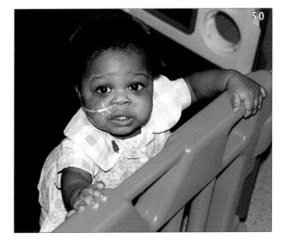

48 i. Nondisjunction (48) occurs in approximately 92–95% of all cases and is attributed to an extra chromosome 21, thus the name 'trisomy 21'. Nondisjunction occurs during meiosis when there is failure of the pair of chromosomes to separate. Mosaicism occurs in approximately 1–3% of cases, when nondisjunction of the 21st chromosome takes place after fertilization. Translocation occurs in approximately 3–6% of cases, when part of chromosome 21 breaks off and attaches to another chromosome.

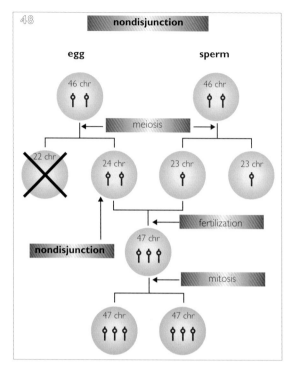

ii. The nurse can offer support to the family and identify appropriate resources for referral. The family's adjustment to the diagnosis will be influenced by the internal family strengths, support from extended family, and the severity of the child's associated problems. One issue for families with a child with Down syndrome is long-range planning for the child's needs.

49 (1) Arrangements can be made for the patient to be at home as much as possible by having nurses come to the home to teach her how to draw blood for laboratory tests and give herself injections of granulocyte colony-stimulating factor. (2) There are small infusion pumps that are packed in a backpack, so that the patient can receive some of her medicine and/or intravenous fluids at home and still spend as much time as possible at home with her children. The nurses would visit the patient to connect the infusion pump.

50 i. The tube is measured from the tip of the nose to the tip of the ear to the xyphoid. Approximately 5–10 cm (2–4 in) is added based on the infant's size. The infant is placed on his right side and the tube is inserted the same as a NG tube.
ii. pH is utilized to confirm nasojejunal placement in many settings. In the jejunum, the pH should be 6.5–7; the pH in the stomach is much more acidic.

51 A male newborn was delivered with exstrophy of the bladder (51).
i. Describe this disorder in the male.
ii. What series of procedures are likely in the staged reconstruction of exstrophy of the bladder suitable for primary closure?

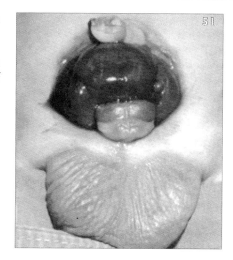

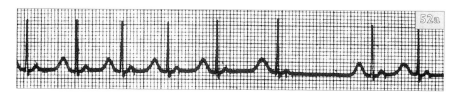

52 A two-year-old, previously healthy male returns home after visiting his grand-parents. His mother notes that he is pale and not acting normally. Concerned, she takes him to the local Emergency Department where his heart rate is 60 beats/min. An EKG (ECG) (52a) is obtained and atrioventricular block is noted. While in the Emergency Department he begins to vomit. The mother is questioned about the possibility of an ingestion and she notes that the grandfather is on 'heart medicine'.
i. What is the diagnosis? What are some of the signs associated with this diagnosis in children?
ii. What does the EKG show?
iii. What are the nursing interventions in the early stages of an acute overdose?
iv. What are other mechanisms of acute cardiac glycoside overdose other than drug ingestion?

51 & 52: Answers

51 i. In this disorder, the posterior portion of the bladder occupying the infra-umbilical area is exposed and the ureteral orifices can be seen. The symphysis pubis and the abdominal wall are widely separated in the midline, while each rectus muscle is attached separately to the ipsilateral pubic bone. Also, the umbilicus is absent. The penis is incomplete and tethered dorsally. The urethra consists of a short strip of mucosa which extends from the bladder to the glans penis. The prepuce is incomplete and ventral in location, while the glans penis is broad and splayed. Although the testes usually are descended, they are associated with inguinal hernias. The scrotum generally is underdeveloped and separated from the penis.
ii. The child will need a series of surgeries, including primary closure of the bladder with or without bilateral ileac osteotomies, bladder neck reconstruction, bilateral ureteral reimplantation, and penile lengthening with single-stage or multistage urethroplasty.

52 i. Acute digitalis intoxication. Common signs of digitalis intoxication in children include sinus bradycardia, ventricular arrhythmias, nausea and vomiting, and hyperkalemia.
ii. The EKG, taken from a child with acute digitalis intoxication, shows atrioventricular block.
iii. Vital sign and EKG monitoring, gastric lavage and decontamination with activated charcoal, monitoring serum digitalis and potassium levels, and administration of the known digitalis antidote drug (Digibind).
iv. Many plant species contain cardiac glycosides. These include: foxglove (52b), common and yellow oleander, lily-of-the-valley, wintersweet, redheaded cottonbush, and pheasant's eye. Ingestion of the leaves, berries, flowers, stems, seeds, or extracts (oils, teas) of these plants can lead to an acute digitalis poisoning. Parents should be able to identify all plants in and around the home, so if a child does ingest a part of the plant it can be readily identified and the proper treatment instituted.

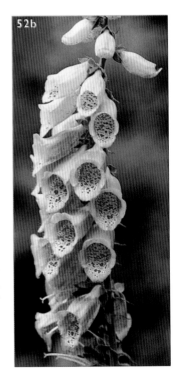
52b

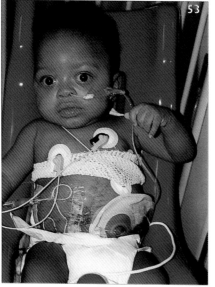

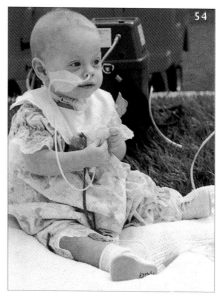

53 This child (53) has had a bowel re-section secondary to NEC. He has an ileostomy and short gut syndrome, and is TPN dependent.

i. What is short gut syndrome, and what does it mean for the child?

When caring for this infant you note that his ostomy is pink and bleeds slight-ly when bag changes are done, and that the skin surrounding the stoma is red and excoriated.

ii. What is your assessment of this situation and the care that must be done?

54 This former premature baby (54) still uses a nasojejunal tube for feedings.

Why is a pacifier attached to her bib?

55 Many parents ask the children's nurse about the need to check their baby's temperature when unwell. Clearly, it is essential for parents not to let their child overheat, nor become hypothermic. Room temperature can play an important part in the overall temperature of a child.

i. What is considered to be the ideal room temperature?

ii. What advice would you give parents about the type of bedding to use?

iii. What information would you give to parents about keeping an unwell baby cool?

53 i. Short gut syndrome refers to the malabsorption and undernutrition after extensive bowel resection, resulting from decreased absorptive surface area, enzyme depletion, and gut hypermotility. Ileal resection is often poorly tolerated because the ileum contains most of the transit sites for nutrient absorption, especially fat, vitamins, and conjugated bile salts. With an ileostomy, rapid bowel transit also occurs. Recovery time for infants with short gut syndrome may take years and recovery potential is related to growth. This infant is subject to many potential problems during this time. They include: potentially life-threatening salt and water losses through the ileostomy; sepsis related to long-term central line and TPN; and TPN-related cholestatic disease (liver dysfunction).

ii. This stoma is normal. A healthy ostomy is dark pink, wet, and shiny. Because the tissue is rich in blood supply, a little bleeding is normal when it is touched. The skin, however, is irritated, possibly because of contact with liquid caustic stool. The appliance must be changed at the first sign of stool leakage. Skin care can be done with water and mild soap, and a skin barrier or ostomy powder may be applied to the skin to decrease irritation. Finally, the appliance opening should be no more than 3 mm (0.125 in) larger than the stoma to minimize contact of stool with the skin.

54 Even though nutrition can be supplied via the nasojejunal tube, infants still need the oral stimulation for sucking and coordinating mouth and tongue motion for future normal feedings. Pacifiers can provide some stimulation and offer some infants the soothing effects via sucking.

55 i. The ideal room temperature is considered to be 18°C (65°F).
ii. Duvets, baby nests, and cot bumpers are not recommended for infants under one year of age. It is advisable to use lightweight blankets that you can adjust to your infant's needs. Below is a guide for parents.
iii. It is important to keep an infant cool when ill, and to contact the family doctor if necessary. There are three important steps to remember:

• Take off layers of bedding/clothing.
• Offer extra fluids, either breast milk, or diluted fruit juices, or water.
• Give antipyretic medications. Always follow the instructions on the bottle carefully.

Room temperature	Amount of bedding to use
15°C (60°F)	Sheet plus four layers of blankets
18°C (65°F)	Sheet plus three to four layers of blankets
21°C (70°F)	Sheet plus two to three layers of blankets
24°C (75°F)	Sheet plus one layer of blanket

56 An 18-year-old, sexually active female is examined for complaints of a genital itch and a copious greenish-yellow discharge. She describes painful urination and a foul-smelling, unpleasant discharge.
i. What are the clinical signs that help differentiate vaginal infections by history?
ii. What kind of infection does she most likely have even before examination?

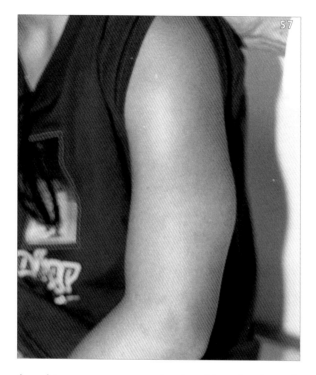

57 When you do a skin assessment you notice that this patient has a firm, egg-shaped swelling of the skin (57) over the area used for the right arm insulin injection. All other injection sites show no evidence of use (e.g. bruising, and needle insertion site marks).
i. What is this abnormality called?
ii. What impact will this have on this patient's blood glucose control?
iii. What do you need to teach the patient in order to correct this problem?

Diagnostic criteria	Normal	Syndrome Bacterial vaginosis	Trichomonas vaginitis	Candida vulvovaginitis
Vaginal pH	3.8–4.2	>4.5	>4.5	<4.5 (usually)
Discharge	White, flocculent	Thin, homogeneous, white, gray, adherent, often increased	Yellow, green, frothy, adherent, increased	White, curdy, 'cottage cheese'-like, sometimes increased
Amine odor (KOH 'whiff' test)	Absent	Present (fishy)	May be present (fishy)	Absent
Main patient complaints	None	Discharge, bad odor, possibly worse after intercourse, itching may be present	Excessive discharge, bad odor, vulvar pruritus, dysuria	Itching/burning, discharge

56 i. Vaginal infections can be differentiated by several observable and reportable characteristics as listed in the table above. They include the physical appearance and the presence or absence of odor or pruritis.
ii. She most likely has a *Trichomonas* infection.

57 i. This raised area is actually fat tissue deposited in response to repeated insulin injections to this site. It is called insulin hypertrophy.
ii. Injecting insulin into an area of hypertrophy may cause delayed insulin absorption. This delayed absorption leads to erratic and unpredictable blood glucose patterns.
iii. This adolescent needs to avoid the raised area entirely and rotate his injection to alternate sites. Gradually, the fatty tissue will disperse and the area may be used once again for injection. Unfortunately, injections given into hypertrophied areas do not hurt and are often favored for that reason. He may be very reluctant to abandon his favorite injection site, and will need encouragement from his parents and the health-care team.

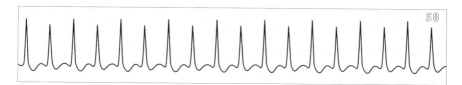

58 A five-day-old male entered the Emergency Department. He was full term, weighed 3.79 kg (8 lb 6 oz), and showed no complications at birth. His parents were concerned about his poor feeding, vomiting, tachypnea, increased sleep, and intermittent irritability. On examination he was difficult to console and he had mild pallor. His skin temperature was slightly cool and he felt clammy. He was alert but appeared tired. He was afebrile with a heart rate of 241 beats/min. An EKG (ECG) (58) was obtained and an intravenous line placed. The baby was diagnosed with SVT.

i. What are the possible precipitating factors of SVT?
ii. What are the signs and symptoms of SVT?
iii. What are the nursing interventions?

59 A nine-month-old male infant with an initial diagnosis of SBS (59) is admitted to the hospital for further observation. Upon stabilization, he is transferred to the Infant Unit where he is a patient for five weeks. During the hospitalization, studies indicate that the child has regressed developmentally, to the age of a two- to three-month-old, and is visually impaired. A gastrostomy tube is placed due to an inability to eat, caused by paralyzed throat muscles, an uncoordinated suck, and no gag reflex. A ventriculoperitoneal shunt is placed due to hydrocephaly and he is diagnosed with a seizure disorder.

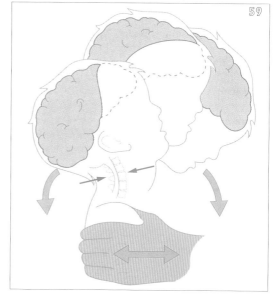

i. Anatomically, why is the infant under one year of age at a higher risk for SBS?
ii. What other laboratory and X-ray studies will likely be ordered after admission to the pediatric ICU, and why?

58 & 59: Answers

58 i. Precipitating factors for SVT include fever, dehydration, fatigue, and exercise. Other factors include caffeine, chocolate, alcohol, cigarettes, and some medications in the older child and adolescent.

ii. The signs and symptoms of SVT include a heart rate >220 beats/min in infants and 150–250 beats/min in children/adolescents. The rhythm is usually regular and the P-wave is unidentifiable. Infants are usually restless and exhibit irritability and poor feeding. They also may have pallor. Children/adolescents exhibit chest pain, pallor, palpitations, and a jittery feeling.

iii. Nursing interventions include assessment and maintenance of the child's airway, breathing, and circulation. Continuous cardiac monitoring and a 12-lead EKG should be in place and available. Intravenous access needs to be obtained for administration of adenosine in a dose of 0.1 mg/kg with a maximum dose 6 mg for the first dose, and maximum of 12 mg for subsequent doses. Propranolol and verapamil are contraindicated in the pediatric population.

59 i. (1) Infants' heads represent approximately 10% of the total body weight versus 2% in the adult. (2) The neck muscles often are much weaker in relation to the body than at other times in life. The weakness of the neck muscles and lack of strong head control mean that more trauma is likely during shaking. (3) Soft cranial sutures and open fontanels leave more room for increased tearing and shearing forces. (4) The infant's brain is unmyelinated, which makes it softer, and thus promotes excessive stretching of the brain and blood vessels, making the brain more susceptible to tearing and shearing. (5) Proportionately larger amounts of CSF in an infant's ventricles and subarachnoid spaces allow the brain to shift farther and faster during vigorous shaking, also increasing stretching and subsequent vessel tears.

ii. (1) CT scan. Subdural and subarachnoid hemorrhage, cerebral edema, and contusions are a result of the tearing of the veins between the outer surfaces of the brain and the inner surfaces of the skull; increased blood within the skull increases the tension and creates the cerebral edema, resulting in high intracranial pressure. (2) Spinal tap. This provides a differentiation between a 'traumatic tap' versus a 'subarachnoid hemorrhage'. If the CSF is initially bloody, and then becomes progressively clearer as it is collected, it is usually due to a traumatic tap (caused by the procedure itself). When the CSF remains bloody, this indicates hemorrhage into the CSF and the cause must be investigated further, with SBS as a possible cause. (3) Skeletal survey. This is to look for previous injuries. It is carried out on the long bones, skull, spine, and ribs, and is done to detect periosteal tears that are associated with SBS, and to identify old and new fractures that indicate previous abuse. (4) Ocular examination. The 'cardinal' sign of SBS is retinal hemorrhages which result from compression of the thorax, high intracranial pressure, and blood flow backwards through the venous channels into the retinal vasculature trees. There may also be orbital/lid ecchymosis, papilledema, subconjunctival hemorrhage, anisocoria, and retinal detachment.

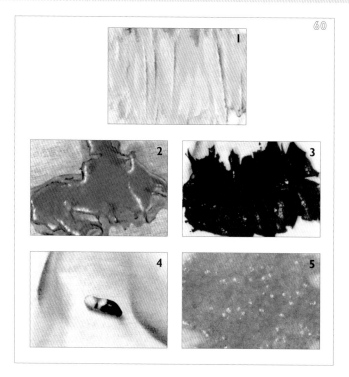

60 Immediately following discharge from the newborn nursery, a male infant's mother phones the hospital with concern that the baby is having gastric difficulty from her breast milk. Although the baby does not seem to be in any discomfort, his stools are loose and pasty.

i. Match the infant stools (60 (1–5)) with their appropriate labels: (a) meconium stool; (b) transitional breast-fed stool; (c) normal breast-fed stool; (d) diarrheal stool; and (e) constipated stool.

ii. If the baby's stool looks like (2), what can the mother be told?

61 A 16-year-old female who is known to be sexually active is seen in the clinic with complaints of fever, lower abdominal tenderness, and dysuria with frequency. Her physical examination reveals adnexal tenderness and cervical motion tenderness. Her laboratory work documents a cervical infection with *Neisseria gonorrhea*.

i. What defines PID?

ii. Should she be admitted to the hospital?

iii. What must the nurse do to help her recover from this episode and teach her how to avoid recurrence?

60 i. The meconium stool is (3); the transitional breast-fed stool is (2); the normal breast-fed stool is (1); the diarrheal stool is (5); and the constipated stool is (4).

ii. Meconial characteristics disappear from the stool gradually in 3–4 days and may be a bit greenish, moist, and poorly formed, with streaks of meconium and light brown mucous threads. The stools gradually become more yellow. The baby is probably fine, undergoing changes in stool that are normal from breast feeding. The baby should generally be observed for any other signs of discomfort or problems with eating if the mother is still concerned.

61 i. According to the CDC, this adolescent demonstrates the minimal criteria and additional evidence to confirm PID:

Criteria	Characteristics
Minimum criteria (plus absence of another established cause)	Lower abdominal tenderness Adnexal tenderness Cervical motion tenderness

Additional criteria (presence of one or more)	Oral temperature >38.3°C (100.94°F)
	Abnormal cervical or vaginal discharge
	Elevated ESR
	Laboratory documentation of cervical infection with
	    Neisseria gonorrhea or Chlamydia trachomatis
	Histopathologic evidence of endometritis on
	    endometrial biopsy
	Tubo-ovarian abscess on sonography or other
	    radiologic tests
	Laparoscopic abnormalities consistent with PID

Possible history	Increased or irregular menstrual flow Cramps Onset of symptoms within one week of menses Dysuria or frequency Partner with recent urethritis

ii. Yes, given the frequency of noncompliance with medical therapy during adolescence and the risk of future reproductive problems, in-patient therapy for adolescents with PID is highly recommended.

iii. In order to help the patient recover from this episode and prevent recurrences of PID, the nurse must be able to communicate effectively. In order to do this, the nurse must understand adolescent development and thought processes to develop rapport in order to offer the support and education the patient needs. The patient must feel comfortable enough to discuss sexual behavior openly in order to be willing and ready to avoid unprotected and unwanted sexual interactions.

62 A 12-year-old male has been admitted to the Emergency Department with an apparent gunshot wound to the chest. His vital signs are poor with a palpable blood pressure of 70 mmHg (9.3 kPa) systolic and a heart rate of 160 beats/min, and it is apparent that he has been hemorrhaging for a while and has lost a lot of blood. Although the paramedics have begun an intravenous infusion, it becomes clear that he needs immediate fluid supplement and will likely need additional vascular access for resuscitative efforts.

i. When should intraosseous infusions be used for vascular access?

ii. What is the best site for initiating an intraosseous infusion, and what are its advantages?

63 A full-term male infant was transferred to the children's hospital at 40 hours of age with a history of abdominal distention. His birth weight was 2.67 kg (5 lb 13 oz) and length 50 cm (19.6 in). His APGAR scores were 9 at 1 minute and 9 at 5 minutes. The infant's abdomen was grossly distended, but he was not in acute distress. He received a series of diatrizoate meglunia (gastrografin) enemas. After the third therapeutic contrast enema, he passed a series of large stools, his abdomen became significantly smaller, and feedings were initiated. He took his feeds eagerly. He continued to stool in small amounts. His sweat test results are shown below.

i. Plot this infant's height and weight on the chart (**63**) and identify the percentile this infant falls within in height and weight.

ii. Based on this infant's history and physical assessment, with what illness are his symptoms most commonly associated?

iii. What information should his parents be taught about his nutritional needs?

iv. What symptoms should mother look for that would indicate a recurrence of bowel obstruction?

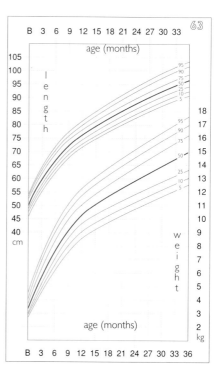

Right side	
Weight	0.1616 mg
Sweat chloride	88.9 mmol/l (mEq/l)*
Left side	
Weight	0.1369 mg
Sweat chloride	89.4 mmol/l (mEq/l)*

*Normal range 0–39.9 mmol/l (mEq/l)

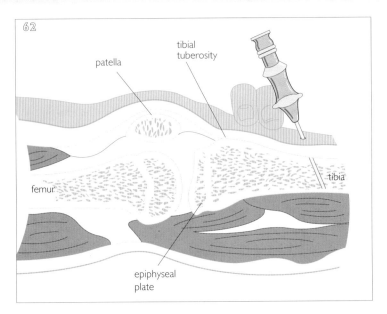

62 i. Intraosseous infusions have become more common, especially when the team has difficulty trying to obtain vascular access by conventional means in children during emergency situations for administration of resuscitative drugs and fluids. It should be reserved as a second line procedure in infants and small children and be used as a temporary means rather than for long-term administration of drugs, blood, or fluids.
ii. Multiple sites have been suggested, including the anterior medial aspect of the tibia, the distal tibia, the distal femur, the sternum, and the ileum. The anterior medial aspect of the tibia (62) is recognized as the site best suited, particularly as it does not interfere with other resuscitative or life-saving measures.

63 i. The infant is in the 50th percentile for height and 5th percentile for weight.
ii. Some 95% of newborns treated for meconium ileus or meconium ileus equivalent are concurrently diagnosed with cystic fibrosis; 20% of children with cystic fibrosis present with meconium ileus at birth.
iii. Cystic fibrosis pancreatic insufficiency is treated with enzyme replacement therapy taken orally with each meal. The quantity of enzymes used varies and is based on the number of calories consumed. Fat-soluble vitamins (A, D, E, K) are administered daily. Supplemental oral salt is necessary during hot weather and periods of prolonged increased sweating.
iv. Complications of meconium ileus occur in about half of such neonates. Symptoms would include: change in stooling pattern, increasing abdominal distention, irritability, abdominal cramping, nausea, vomiting, and loss of interest in feeding.

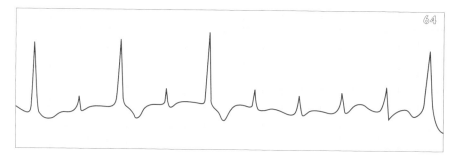

64 This EKG (ECG) (**64**) tracing is from a 10-week-old, male infant who was admitted to the pediatric unit with retractions, tachypnea, and hypothermia. He was born prematurely to an HIV-positive mother. Shortly after admission, a central line was established to provide nutrition. *Pneumocystis carinii* pneumonia was ruled out; however, he was treated for a fungal sepsis. He developed premature ventricular contractions after the therapy was completed, blood gases were normal, and X-ray confirmed proper placement of the central line. The dysrhythmia abated after treatment with lidocaine and he was discharged after 10 more weeks of hospitalization. What could the PVCs be attributed to?

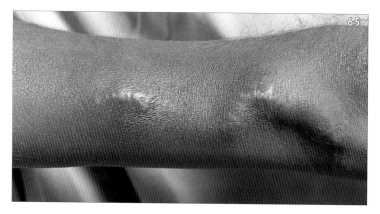

65 i. What is represented here (**65**)? What would this be used for?
ii. What complications do nurses need to assess for when taking care of a child with this technology?
iii. Why is it important to teach an adolescent who has this type of vascular access site?

64 & 65: Answers

64 The PVCs were most likely from HIV myocarditis since alternative explanations for the dysrhythmia were ruled out and the problem abated.

65 i. An AV fistula which is used as an internal access site for hemodialysis.
ii. Three major complications that nurses need to assess for are:

- Patency. It is important for the nurse to assess the patency of the AV fistula before using it, auscultating the fistula for a bruit, and its quality and intensity. A diminished sound could be indicative of fibrin formation, and would require further evaluation by the physician.
- Infection. Assess the area for signs of erythema, edema, pain, or drainage. The presence of any of these factors would indicate the need for a further assessment to be made to see if the site is infected. If drainage is present, a culture of the drainage is necessary. Follow-up with the physician is also indicated.
- Pseudoaneurysm/aneurysm. Observe vascular access site for signs of bulging. Prevention of this complication is the goal, and rotation of sites during needle insertion can help to minimize this complication. The physician must be informed if an aneurysm is observed.

iii. It is important that the patient be knowledgeable about preventive methods for protecting the AV fistula access. This is accomplished by, first, teaching the adolescent to protect the patency of the site:

- Not to wear restrictive, tight clothing or jewelry around any affected extremity.
- Not to apply a lot of pressure to the site (i.e. do not allow the blood pressure to be taken on the extremity with vascular access).
- Not to put a lot of weight on the site, especially for an extended period of time (i.e. do not sleep on top of the arm with vascular access).
- Avoid contact sports that could lead to the site being hit or injured.
- Avoid bending the limb with the access site for extended periods of time, in order to prevent cutting off adequate blood flow through the fistula.

Secondly, teach the patient to monitor the site for signs of infection (this is not as prevalent with internal access sites, but has been reported):

- Observe the site daily for any signs of redness, swelling, pain, or drainage. Report any observations immediately.
- Instruct the patient about the necessity of reporting any pain or discomfort in the area to the nurse providing his/her care.

66 A three-year-old male who has been seen on frequent occasions in the child health clinic is below the predicted percentile for his height. His mother complains that he is 'frequently off-color' with nonspecific-type illness. He has no specific symptoms.
i. What is a possible diagnosis for this child?
ii. What nursing interventions should be performed?
iii. What is the significance of UTI, what further investigations should be undertaken, and why are they important?

67 A nine-year-old female with a long history of asthma comes to the school nurse's office. She is clutching her throat and indicating she is having trouble breathing, is crying, and appears fearful. Your immediate concern is that she is choking, but she keeps pointing to her chest and when you ask if she has asthma, she shakes her head, yes. You listen to her chest. No wheezing and minimal breath sounds are heard. She is on a salbuterol (salbutamol; Albuterol) MDI and a sodium cromoglycate (cromolyn; Intal) inhaler, but has neither of these at school today.

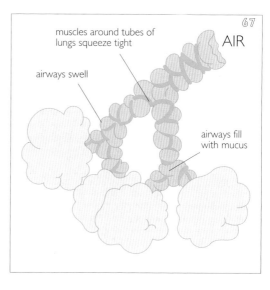

Protocols at school allow you to start treatment for her, including two puffs of salbuterol from the clinic supply of MDIs via a spacing device, followed in 3–4 minutes with two puffs of sodium cromoglycate. When you assess her chest again you are able to hear sparse wheezing throughout her chest, but air exchange remains compromised.

Standing orders allow you to give two aerosol treatments, 20 minutes apart, with 0.5 ml salbuterol and 2 ml sodium cromoglycate. You administer these treatments to her. Each time you listen to her chest she has increased wheezing throughout and mild improvement in her air exchange. However, after her last treatment she is unable to get above 260 l/min on the peak flow meter and her lungs are still not clear.

Based on the drawing of lungs before an asthma attack (**67**):
i. What signs and symptoms result from lung changes during an acute asthma episode?
ii. What should your next action be?

66 i. Failure to thrive may be the result of numerous causes; however, a less obvious cause may be due to chronic undetected UTI. This possible cause must be excluded if no other diagnosis is made.

ii. Obtaining a specimen of urine either by clean catch technique, or by using a urine collection pad, is essential to facilitate microscopic examination (either in the ward environment or laboratory) before starting appropriate antibiotic treatment. This will also establish a diagnosis of UTI. However, a child who has had previous asymptomatic UTIs (and sustained renal damage) may not have an active UTI when a random specimen of urine is taken.

The vigilant pediatric nurse should be aware that the child may have had a previously undiagnosed UTI and should encourage discussion with the multidisciplinary team about the possibility of previous renal damage. It is also advisable to facilitate the organization of appropriate renal investigations.

iii. UTI in childhood is common, with approximately 3% of children affected. UTI in conjunction with VUR can cause permanent renal damage. Though most children do not have sequelae, some develop scars which can extend with further infections.

Hypertension develops in over 20% of patients with scars, and up to 10% may develop end-stage renal failure, often many years later. Some 20% of all kidney transplants performed at any age in the UK are because of scars caused by childhood UTIs. Scarring can only be initiated by UTIs in early childhood, and can occur very quickly after only a few days' infection.

Establishing a diagnosis of UTI can be very difficult in young children, as symptoms are often vague and nonspecific. An awareness of the possibility of a previously undetected UTI causing significant renal scarring may be an important cause of failure to thrive.

Renal damage should be excluded in a child with 'failure to thrive' if no other diagnosis is established. The child should be investigated regardless of age or gender. Investigations should include an abdominal ultrasound scan to exclude gross anatomical abnormalities and a DMSA radioisotope scan to exclude renal scarring.

In a child under one year of age, a micturating cystogram may be performed to exclude VUR.

67 i. An acute asthma episode will usually manifest itself with wheezing or a persistent, harsh dry cough. Some individuals wheeze, some cough, and some do both. Sometimes, when early warning signs are not noticed, the bronchospasm can be severe enough that chest assessment reveals no wheezing and minimal air exchange is heard, hence a silent chest. Children need repeated education about asthma in order to recognize when an attack is beginning and how to deal with this.

ii. An ambulance should be called and the child transported to the nearest emergency facility. She is now stabilized and has some air exchange established; however, she needs additional treatment and monitoring under a physician's care. Her parents should be notified that she is being transported, where she is being sent, and why. Notify her family physician of this acute episode.

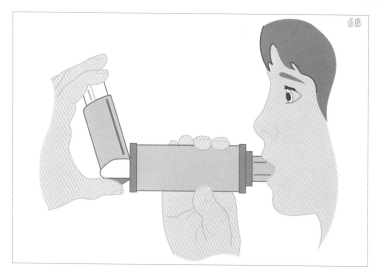

68 With regard to the case in **67**:
i. What can trigger an acute asthma episode?
ii. Why are salbuterol (salbutamol; Albuterol) and sodium cromoglycate (cromolyn; Intal) often given to asthma patients in combination with each other?
iii. Why are spacing devices like the one illustrated (**68**) important to use with children?
iv. What other drug could be added to the patient's regimen at this time to reduce swelling and prolong the intervals between acute episodes?

69 This one-month-old infant (**69**) has Trisomy 18. It is the second most frequent autosomal disorder and occurs with a prevalence of 1 in 4,000 to 1 in 5,000 live-born infants.
i. What are the distinguishing features?
ii. Most of these infants die at approximately one year of age. What is the cause?

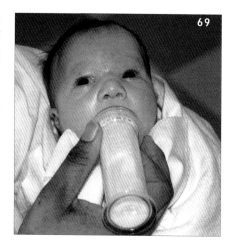

68 & 69: Answers

68 i. An asthma 'trigger' is any substance an asthmatic comes in contact with that causes symptoms of wheezing, coughing, and difficulty with breathing. Common asthma 'triggers' include – but are not limited to – the following items: pollens (grass, trees, flowers, and weeds); cigarette and cigar smoke; dust and dust mites; cockroaches; mold and mildew; viral infections; inhalants (chemical or cleaning products, and perfume); allergens (certain foods, feathers, and animal dander); changes in the weather and air pollution; and exercise. Children need to learn what their specific 'triggers' are, and how to avoid or minimize contact with them. Parents need to learn housekeeping techniques that decrease 'triggers' at home and in their immediate environment.

ii. Salbutarol is a bronchodilator that can be inhaled directly into the lungs. It acts to decrease the bronchospasm and permits air exchange to occur. Side-effects of salbutarol include tachycardia, palpitations, and irritability. Sodium cromoglycate is an inhaled anti-inflammatory agent used in the preventive management of asthma. Consistent use over time should decrease the number and severity of asthma episodes. During an acute asthma attack, not only does bronchospasm occur, but there is also inflammation of the mucous membrane lining the bronchial tree, as well as increased mucus production. Sodium cromoglycate is used to prevent asthma episodes from occurring as frequently, and to reduce some of the inflammation in the bronchial tree. It is not an antihistamine, however. Side-effects of sodium cromoglycate are rare.

iii. The speed of medication bursting forth from an inhaler has been measured as high as 65 mph (105 kph). For a child to coordinate his/her breathing with that speed of medication delivery is difficult. The medication ends up on the soft palate or the back of the throat, and not in the lungs. A spacer is an enclosed chamber in which the inhaler fits on one end and a mask or mouthpiece on the other end. Once the mask or mouthpiece is in place, it becomes a closed system. Medication can then be delivered directly into the spacer and inhaled without being lost or wasted.

iv. Prednisone, given intramuscularly or orally, helps to reverse a severe asthma episode. Usually, oral prednisone is prescribed for 5–10 days following a severe, acute asthma episode. With children who are chronic and severe asthmatics, inhaled steroids are often added to their daily regimen of treatment. Inhaled steroids do not have the unwanted side-effects of oral steroids because they are inhaled directly into the lungs and do not circulate throughout the system. Anyone using an inhaled steroid needs to rinse out their mouth after use. Inhaled steroids tend to encourage the growth of oral *Candida*, which can be an unpleasant side-effect. Adults on long-term inhaled steroids have shown a greater incidence in the development of glaucoma.

69 i. Prenatal growth deficiency, microcephaly, small face, prominent occiput, high nasal bridge, palpebral fissures, small mouth, overriding fingers, camptodactyly, clenched hand, and hypoplastic nails are characteristic of Trisomy 18.

ii. Ninety per cent of these infants die because of cardiac or central nervous system malformation or respiratory infection. The exact reason for decreased survivability is not always known. The few individuals who have survived into adolescence have marked mental retardation.

Glasgow Coma Scale	Score	Pediatric scale	Score
Eye opening			
Spontaneous	4		
To speech	3	Same as adult scale	
To pain	2		
None	1		
Best verbal response			
Oriented	5	Coos, babbles	5
Confused	4	Irritable cry	4
Inappropriate words	3	Cries to pain	3
Incomprehensible sounds	2	Moans to pain	2
None	1	None	1
Best motor response			
Obeys commands	6	Normal spontaneous movement	6
Localizes pain	5	Withdraws to touch	5
Withdraws	4	Withdraws to pain	4
Flexion posturing	3	Abnormal flexion	3
Extensor posturing	2	Abnormal extension	2
None	1	None	1

70 A 15-year-old male has been admitted from the Emergency Department following a motor vehicle crash. The youth was an unrestrained front-seat passenger in a 1990 model small car. On arrival at the Emergency Department, he opened his eyes to noxious stimuli. He would cry, 'Mama help me', repeatedly, but not answer questions. He pushed away when the nurse attempted to pass a NG tube. He has facial lacerations and a 'boggy' left anterior skull.
i. What is his GCS score?
ii. What will be the priorities for care?
iii. What additional information will need to be collected over the next 60 hours?

71 A seven-year-old male has three months to go before he completes his therapy for acute lymphocytic leukemia. He is in clinic today for his monthly visit and his father reports one testicle is larger than the other.
i. How can the orchidometer (71) be used to determine testicular size?
ii. What other question could you ask the child and his father to determine if this is leukemia infiltrate?

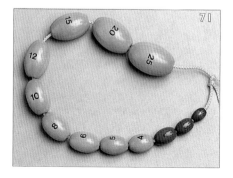

70 i. GCS provides a standardized system to assess cerebral function. For preverbal children, there is a modified scale. The adolescent would score a 2 to eye opening since he opens his eyes to noxious stimuli. He does not answer questions and his verbalization is understandable, but out of context, scoring a 4 in verbal response. Since he can localize the nurse and noxious stimuli of the NG tube, he would score a 5 for motor response. His total score is 11. Changes in the total or subscale score over time should be tracked and reported. A GCS score of <8 following resuscitation is indicative of severe head injuries.

ii. Priorities for trauma care are airway, breathing, and circulation. His airway should be evaluated for patency and supported if compromised. A part of airway management is cervical spine stabilization. The cervical spine should be immobilized manually or with properly fitted immobilization devices. Once the airway is secured, breathing function must be evaluated. Adequate rate and depth of ventilation is particularly important with head injury to reduce cerebral edema. The next priority is to address circulation. Hemorrhagic shock must be corrected. Adequate intravascular volume is necessary to maintain cerebral perfusion. If the required volume replacement is >60 ml/kg, whole blood should be used for subsequent boluses. Airway, breathing, and circulation are re-evaluated frequently as the evaluation process continues. The next priority is to evaluate the degree of neurologic disability. All efforts to prevent secondary brain injury due to expansion of intracranial volume are initiated, including supporting ventilation, maintaining cerebral perfusion, and reducing metabolic demands. Once airway, breathing, circulation, and disability are addressed, a secondary survey of all body systems must be completed to reveal any other injuries and determine a definitive plan of care.

iii. Serial evaluation of breathing, circulation, and neurologic disability is critical to identifying progression or stabilization of injury over time. Vital signs should include heart rate, blood pressure, respiratory rate, end-tidal carbon dioxide, pulse oximetry, and intracranial pressure if a device is inserted. Clinical evaluation of aeration, capillary refill time, and pulse volumes are also helpful in evaluating respiratory and circulatory status. Serial scoring with the GCS and reflex examination will provide useful information about the progression of neurologic function. Other causes of altered mental status must also be ruled out using a drug screen and blood alcohol level.

71 i. Use the orchidometer by selecting the wooden model which is closest in size to the testicle determined by palpation.

ii. Is there pain in either testicle? Leukemia infiltrate results in painless enlargement of one or both testicles.

Motion	Right hip	Left hip
Abduction	20°	45°
Adduction	10°	20°
External rotation	50°	40°
Internal rotation	−20°	15°
Flexion	80°	120°
Figure-four sign	Positive	Negative

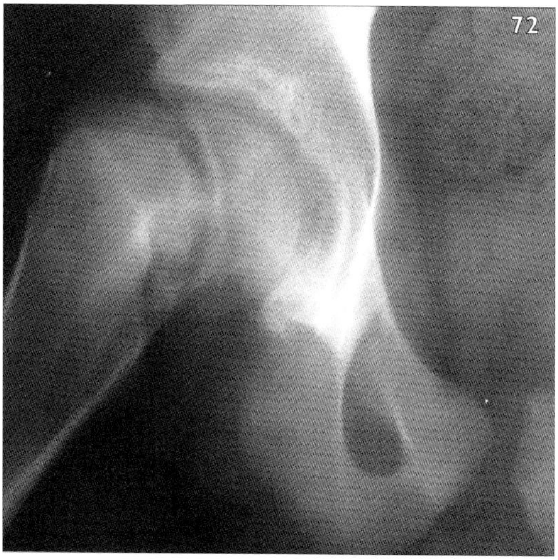

72 A 13-year-old, obese black male presents with a one-day history of right groin and thigh pain. He walks with a severe painful limp, keeping his right foot in external rotation. On the previous day, he was tackled while playing football. Upon hitting the ground he experienced a sharp pain in the right groin. Physical examination reveals the results shown above. X-rays were taken of both hips (**72**).

i. After reviewing the patient's history, physical examination, and X-rays, what is the diagnosis?
ii. What is the usual medical treatment for this problem? What should you tell the parent and adolescent about caring for him before surgery?
iii. What are the possible complications that may result from this problem?
iv. What is the likelihood that this problem will occur in the opposite hip? What is the best prevention to avoid recurrence?

73 i. What sequelae are often associated with SBS?
ii. On discharge, what referrals and follow-up should be made in order to support a family caring for their SBS child?

72 i. The patient has the classic signs of a slipped capital femoral epiphysis:

- High-risk group: obese, black, male.
- Age group: adolescents (males 13–15 years, before growth plates are closed).
- Characteristic pain: groin, thigh, or knee.
- History of trauma: often precedes an acute or unstable slip.
- Range of motion: all but external rotation on affected side decreased. Patient typically walks with foot in internal rotation. When hip and knee are flexed, the leg rotates externally into a figure-four sign. No external rotation of the hip can be elicited.
- X-rays: indicate the femoral neck has slipped anteriorly and upwards on the femoral head through the growth plate.

ii. The patient requires a surgical pinning of the right hip as soon as possible. Occasionally, a severely displaced acute or unstable slip will require traction prior to surgery to reduce it. Until the patient undergoes surgery, he/she will be on crutches and nonweight-bearing on the affected side.

iii. (1) Chondrolysis: a deterioration of the cartilage of the hip joint. (2) Avascular necrosis: loss of circulation to the femoral head. The patient should be monitored for these complications for six months following surgery.

iv. This patient has a 25% chance of having this problem occur in the opposite hip. The only way the patient may decrease this chance is by losing weight.

73 i. Approximately one-third of infants suffer little or no sequelae; one-third experience permanent brain damage, developmental delay, blindness, seizures, and paralysis; and one-third of infants die. SBS carries significant morbidity and mortality and is frequently associated with intellectual impairment and permanent brain damage, as well as developmental delay, spasticity, quadraparesis, hearing loss, hydrocephalus, seizures, microcephaly, and blindness.

ii. Referrals:

- Child Protective Services (once diagnosis is suspected) mandatory.
- Rehabilitative Services for the child (physical, occupational, speech).
- Family counseling services, mandatory.
- Parenting classes, mandatory.
- Services for hearing and visual impairment.

Follow-up:

- Primary health care physician.
- Physical, occupational, and speech therapy.
- Neurology and gastroenterology.

Resources:

- Charity organizations specializing in special-case infants (e.g. in the USA, March of Dimes).
- Cerebral Palsy Foundation.
- State and County specific resources (e.g. early intervention and special education).

74 A 15-year-old female who is sexually active and on oral contraceptives telephones to ask advice about her pills. She forgot to take her pills and wants to know if she needs additional contraceptive protection.
i. What questions should you ask, and what advice would you give regarding back-up method?
ii. How should she restart her pills?

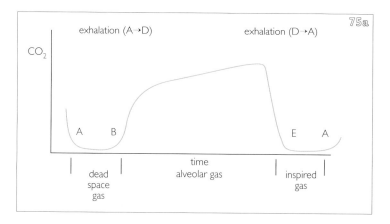

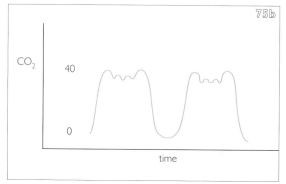

75 A critically ill 18-month-old male infant with respiratory failure is intubated, given a chemical paralyzing agent, and placed on a ventilator. His end-tidal CO_2 is monitored by a capnometer.
i. Describe the capnogram shown in (75a).
ii. What does this infant's capnogram (75b) indicate?

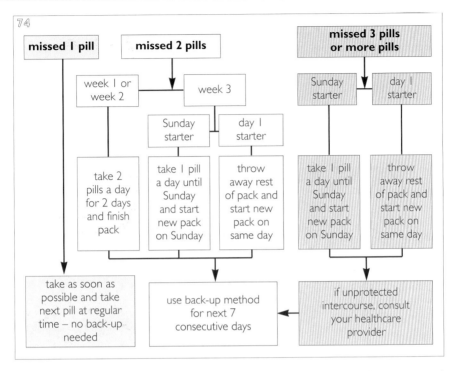

74 i. It is important to know the specifics of the girl's missed pills – how many and whether they are in week 1, 2, or 3 of her menstrual cycle. If she missed one pill, she should take it right away and no back-up is necessary. If two pills were forgotten in the first, second or third weeks, she should use back-up method for the next seven consecutive days. If three pills or more were missed, and if she has had unprotected intercourse, she should consult her primary physician and use back-up method for the next seven consecutive days.

ii. Depending on when she missed her pills and how many she missed, she should follow the guidelines in (74).

75 i. The pediatric capnometer provides a numerical display of the end-tidal CO_2 with a capnogram that is a graphic recording of waveform produced by changes in the level of exhaled CO_2 over the respiratory cycle. 75a is a fast-speed (25 mm/s) capnogram of a single respiratory cycle. The vertical axis represents CO_2 concentration; the horizontal axis indicates time.

ii. Partial neuromuscular blockade or return of voluntary respiratory function will be first seen in capnograms as a cleft in the alveolar plateau (75b). This is caused by the rush of CO_2-free gas into the lungs as the diaphragm contracts. It can indicate early signs that more paralyzing agent is needed.

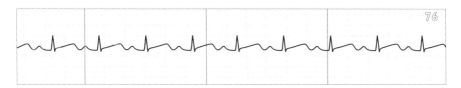

76 This EKG (ECG) tracing (76) is from a four-month-old, female infant who was hospitalized for fever and tachypnea. This infant's other symptoms included retractions and nasal flaring. Both parents were HIV positive. The child was found to have *Pneumocystis carinii* pneumonia and cytomegalovirus infection. A presumptive diagnosis of AIDS was made. She was started on intravenous antibiotic treatment, but the condition worsened and the child became progressively hypoxemic requiring increased FIO_2 and eventual intubation with mechanical ventilation.

The PR interval for this age and heart rate is 0.12 seconds. This EKG strip showed a PR interval of 0.16 seconds and a heart rate of 136 beats/min. What is her cardiac status and prognosis?

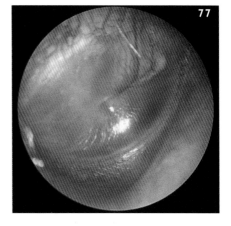

77 A two-year-old male, seen by the primary physician for evaluation of an upper respiratory infection which had been present for five days, is now complaining of bilateral otalgia (ear pain) and a low-grade fever. His mother feels that he has also been less responsive to her for the past week. After a complete evaluation the child was diagnosed with a bilateral otitis media and placed on oral antibiotics.

i. What clinical signs may be present in a child with an acute otitis media with effusion?

A healthy tympanic membrane in the right ear is shown (77).

ii. What otoscopic findings of an infected ear are not illustrated?

iii. What are the other causes of otalgia?

iv. What are the potential complications of acute otitis media?

v. Other than a tympanic membrane perforation, what other disease processes present with otorrhea (ear discharge)?

76 The EKG strip, family history, and clinical presentation suggests first-degree heart block caused by HIV myocarditis. The infant's condition was poor and she died three weeks after admission.

77 i. Clinical signs that may be present in a child with an acute otitis media are multiple and each child should be evaluated on an individual basis, including a complete physical examination. These include:

- Otalgia, which may be unilateral or bilateral.
- Fever, which may or may not be present.
- Decreased hearing caused by the accumulation of fluid behind the tympanic membrane.
- Otorrhea, which requires further evaluation of the source, i.e. possible tympanic membrane perforation with a secondary otitis externa.
- Vertigo.
- Tinnitus.
- Nausea/vomiting.
- Anorexia.
- Associated URI.
- Inconsolability.
- Crying, often greater when the child is in the supine position.
- Behavioral changes.
- Pulling at the ears.
- Popping sounds in the ears.

ii. Otoscopic findings include: erythematous (red) tympanic membrane, no visualization of landmarks, may be pus filled, and no mobility with pneumotoscopy.

iii. Otalgia may also be referred pain from some other origin such as teething, pharyngitis, tonsillitis, dental caries, oral trauma, and oral lesions associated with viral illnesses.

iv. The complications of an otitis media include:

- Tympanic membrane perforation.
- Hearing loss.
- Sepsis (greater occurrence in the neonatal population).
- Meningitis.
- Intracranial/extracranial abscess.
- Facial nerve paralysis.
- Mastoiditis.
- Sigmoid sinus thrombosis.
- Otitic hydrocephalus.

v. Other disease processes that may involve otorrhea are cholesteatoma, otitis externa, foreign body in ear, ear canal wall trauma, and seborrheic dermatitis. Cerumen has also been mistaken for otorrhea, given its many variations of normal.

78 With regard to the boy in 77, what nursing interventions should be done with the parent?

79 A four-year old male presents with an L4–L5 level myelomeningocele. He has several bowel movements a day that are usually small and hard, though occasionally he has large liquid stools. Currently he is not on a program for bowel management. The child also has a neurogenic bladder that is managed by clean intermittent catheterization done four times each day and taking oxybutynin hydrochloride (Ditropan). The mother mentions that the family is planning a vacation to a beach in a warm climate in the near future.

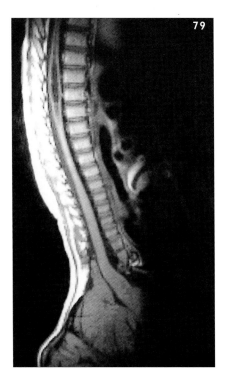

i. The patient's MRI scan (79) reveals a syrinx in the thoracic spinal cord. What signs/symptoms of a symptomatic spinal cord syrinx should the parents be taught to observe for?

ii. Liquid stools may be caused by a variety of reasons such as bacterial infections, viral infections, or medications. What other reason might make a child with a myelomeningocele have liquid stools ?

iii. What teaching should done with the parents to prevent problems from occurring during the family's upcoming vacation?

78 Nursing interventions should include teaching the parent specific instructions on taking the prescribed antibiotic medication including dosage, frequency, and duration. Compliance with taking the amount of antibiotic prescribed at the right time for the full duration should be stressed. If the child has not improved within 48–72 hours after starting the medication (i.e. sustained fever), re-evaluation by the family doctor is recommended. A mild analgesic may be given for pain or discomfort the child may be experiencing. Dosage should be calculated for each child (given their weight in kg) so that optimal pain relief will be achieved. The use of antihistamines and decongestants play no role in the resolution of an otitis media; however, they are useful in reducing nasal congestion associated with URI. If any complications (as above) should present, immediate medical attention should be sought. Follow-up evaluation with the physician is recommended at three to four weeks following diagnosis of the infection, provided the child remains asymptomatic. Reassure the parents that the current hearing loss is probably temporary, due to the fluid accumulation in the middle ear space. If there are concerns following resolution of the middle ear effusion, an audiogram is recommended.

79 i. A change in bowel or bladder function, weakness of the upper extremities, a change in gait or ambulatory endurance, or a worsening of scoliosis are possible symptoms of a spinal cord syrinx.
ii. Children with an L4–L5 myelomeningocele are prone to fecal impactions which may be so severe that only liquid stool is able to be expelled past the obstruction.
iii. Due to the fact that the child is on oxybutynin hydrochloride – which may decrease the ability of the child to sweat – the parents need to be instructed to protect the child from heat exhaustion. The parents should be instructed to monitor the child and ensure he has an adequate intake of liquids and takes frequent rest periods during the day. The parents also need to be aware that adequate sunblock should be applied prior to sun exposure, as insensate skin may become severely burned without causing pain. The child with an L4–L5 myelomeningocele has decreased sensation in the lower extremities and may not feel any pain when trauma or injury to their feet occurs. Therefore, the family should make sure that the child wears protective footwear at all times, even on the beach or while swimming. They should also inspect the child's feet at least once a day to ensure that no trauma to the feet has occurred.

80 This female infant (80) is five days old, and her parents are white European in origin. In assessing an infant the color and texture of the skin provide a range of details, that may lead to further examination by the medical team.

i. Describe briefly assessment of a new-born infant's skin.

ii. This baby has a rash, what may be the cause?

iii. Give a definition of a post-term infant.

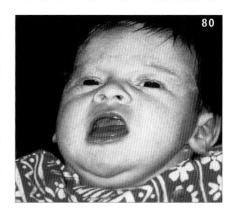

81 This particular type of gastrostomy tube (81) is surgically inserted to provide nutrition. Name or describe the parts of the tube labeled 1–7.

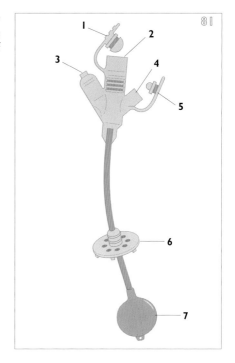

82 What would be the first line of treatment for a child known to be allergic to a specific substance presenting with signs of anaphylaxis?

80–82: Answers

80 i. You will want to ensure that the baby is laid in a safe and warm position to undertake your assessment. In the majority of infants from white ethnic groups you will find that they present with pale skin over the body. However, their hands and feet may be slightly blue for the first 24–48 hours. Any indication of central cyanosis, an unusual pallor, or jaundice warrants further investigation. For infants with a darker skin it is important to examine the mucous membranes of the mouth to assess for pallor. In babies of mixed race the racial coloring may not be immediately obvious; however, in male infants the scrotum is often pigmented. You should note any birth marks.

ii. The superficial peeling of skin, particularly over the extremities, is fairly common during the first week of life. This occurs commonly in post-term (postmature) babies or those who have suffered from intrauterine malnutrition. There is no specific treatment.

iii. A post-term infant is one born after more than 41 weeks' gestation.

81 The parts are:

1 The feeding port cover.
2 The feeding port is where liquid nourishment enters the tube via a delivery system that is connected to the feeding port.
3 The balloon port is typically a hard plastic valve where water or saline can be inserted to inflate the balloon located near the tip of the gastrostomy tube.
4 The medication port can be used to deliver liquid medication during continuous feeding.
5 The medication port cover seals the port.
6 The external ring holds the tube securely in the proper position. It may be sutured to the skin to prevent the tube from moving, ensuring that the tract will heal properly.
7 The retention balloon contains water or saline to hold the tube inside the stomach.

82 After immediately summoning for a paramedic ambulance, the first line of treatment for anaphylaxis is the administration of an adrenaline autoinjector device, given directly into the outer thigh. This device must be given without delay, so the parents or caregivers of children known to be at risk must always carry the prescribed adrenaline at all times. Following a careful and detailed medical assessment, usually undertaken at a specialist allergy center, the device most commonly prescribed is EpiPen. This is a user friendly, autoinjector concealing a spring-activated, concealed needle. The EpiPen delivers the adrenaline quickly and efficiently. It is able to be given through clothing and has a two-year shelf life. Adrenaline acts quickly to constrict the blood vessels, relaxing the smooth muscles in the lungs to improve breathing. The heartbeat is stimulated and any severe swelling around the face, mouth, and lips (angioedema) is reduced.

83 A young female adolescent is in the clinic for her routine 10-year-old check-up. Her height is 140 cm (55 in) and her weight is 56 kg (124 lb).
i. What method might be used to assess degree of obesity using height and weight?
ii. Why is this formula used?

84 A two-year-old boy fell as the result of jumping on a bed, and he sustained a left femur fracture. He was admitted to the hospital and placed into Bryant's traction for two days (84a), then placed in a spica cast for discharge (84b).
i. What is the purpose of Bryant's traction?
ii. What assessment and nursing interventions are pertinent in relation to skin care for a child in Bryant's traction?
iii. What signs of complications should be noted in a child in a spica cast?

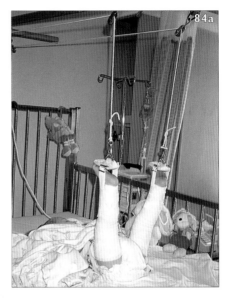

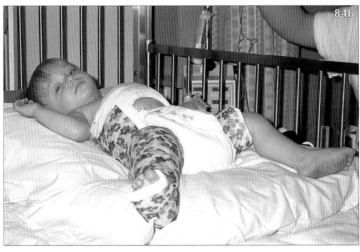

83 i. The BMI formula is considered to be a reliable indicator of degree of obesity. A BMI factor over 30 would suggest referral for further assessment and treatment.

ii. This formula is considered easy to use, requiring only a height and weight measurement with a short mathematical calculation, and it has correlation with body fat assessment.

Calculation: $$\frac{\text{Weight (kg)}}{\text{Height (m)}^2} = \text{BMI} \qquad \text{or} \qquad \frac{\text{Weight (lb)}}{\text{Height (in)}^2} \times 750 = \text{BMI}$$

BMI	Description
≤20	Underweight
20–25	Desirable
25–30	Overweight
30–40	Morbidly/severely obese

84 i. Bryant's traction is a type of running skin traction used on children under two years of age, weighing between 12–14 kg (26.5–31 lb). The traction pulls the legs upward, stretching the muscles around the fracture, thus allowing for easier alignment of the fracture.

ii. The 'ace wraps' should be removed two to three times a day to prevent circulatory compromise and skin break down. The skin should be inspected for any areas of redness or irritation. If the skin is intact, alcohol or witch-hazel should be applied to toughen the skin. Powders and lotions should never be used. Powder builds up around the edges of the 'ace wraps'; lotions soften the skin, leading to irritation. Extra attention should be given to the skin over bony prominences such as the ankle and coccyx.

iii. Circulatory compromise could be indicated by a change in color or temperature in the toes, or numbness and tingling which does not go away after changing the child's position. A foul odor, moisture from the cast, a temperature of 101°C (50°F) lasting more than one day, or unusual irritability could all be indicative of an infection. A sudden increase in pain with a change in neurovascular assessment could be a sign of compartment syndrome.

85 This child (85) was diagnosed at birth with Down syndrome. Down syndrome is associated with a recognizable phenotype and limited intellectual capacity because of extra chromosome 21 material.

i. What facial characteristics are associated with Down syndrome?

ii. What other associated problems are seen with Down syndrome?

iii. What is the nurse's role in primary care management of the child with Down syndrome?

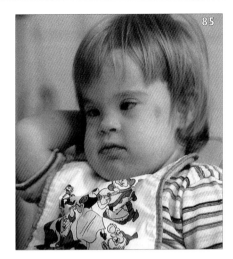

86 A four-year-old male is brought into the clinic with the chief complaint of a persistent URI for two weeks. He has had persistent rhinorrhea, which is clear to purulent in nature. He is unable to sleep at night due to coughing. His appetite has also been decreased. After a complete evaluation he was then diagnosed with an acute sinusitis.

One of the diagnostic tests used in the work-up of a child with a chronic sinusitis is the CT scan.

i. In the illustration (86), which of the maxillary sinuses is affected?

ii. What nursing interventions should be implemented?

iii. What are the potential complications of a sinus infection?

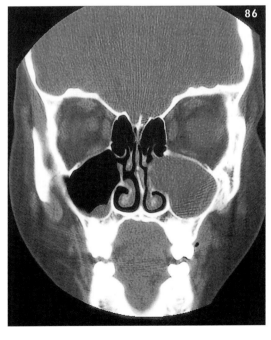

iv. What populations are at higher risk of recurrent–chronic sinusitis?

85 i. The most common facial features seen in this child are: epicanthic folds; strabismus; reduced interorbital distance; small, low-set and shortened ears; flat nasal bridge; and prominent, thickened, and fissured lips. The mouth is typically held open and the tongue is often enlarged and protruding.

ii. Upper respiratory problems, as well as pneumonia, are common in Down syndrome children. Other associated problems include: cardiac anomalies; mental retardation; gastrointestinal tract anomalies; growth retardation and obesity; visual and hearing abnormalities; musculoskeletal/motor dysfunction; altered immune system; dental/oral motor problems; thyroid dysfunction; leukemia and seizure disorders.

iii. The nurse's role is to coordinate and assist the parents in managing the health care and educational systems. Primary care management includes: diet; safety; immunizations; monitoring growth and development; screening (vision, hearing, dental, blood pressure, hematocrit, urinalysis, tuberculosis, thyroid function, hip dislocations, and mitral valve prolapse).

86 i. The left side, with a thickening of the base of the right side of the maxillary sinus. Symptoms of an acute sinusitis include persistent rhinorrhea for >10 days, with no improvement of the symptoms during that time. Consistency of the rhinorrhea has no bearing on the diagnosis of an infection, and it can be clear, white, or yellow/green in nature. Rhinorrhea associated with a viral illness may also present, but usually clears by 10 days. Other symptoms include daytime/nocturnal cough, halitosis, fever may/may not be present, headaches, periorbital edema, and behavioral changes. Facial pain may also be present, but is very subjective. Children do experience 'head pain', that may be manifested by irritability, fussiness, and pulling on their hair and ears.

ii. The nurse should stress the importance of compliance with the antibiotic therapy given. (A 21-day course or seven days past the resolution of symptoms is recommended.) A mild analgesic may be given for discomfort. Decongestants can also be given for systematic relief. Aspirin is not recommended for more than three days. Normal saline nasal sprays can be used liberally to help thin secretions. Mucolytics can also be used. The use of antihistamines is discouraged as they may result in thickened secretions. Follow-up evaluation is recommended.

iii. Potential complications include intraorbital abscess, periorbital cellulitis, intracranial abscess, visual loss, meningitis, and cavernous sinus thrombosis. Parents should be taught to observe for signs and symptoms indicating that they need to see a health care provider immediately should any of these occur. These include continued or increased signs of infection, or changes in neurologic status.

iv. High-risk populations include patients with craniofacial abnormalities, cystic fibrosis, mechanical obstruction (e.g. choanal atresia, deviated septum, choncha bullosa), immotile cilia syndrome, immunodeficiency, and gastroesophageal reflux. Other conditions associated with sinusitis include patients with adenoid hypertrophy, nasal foreign body, or sinonasal tumors.

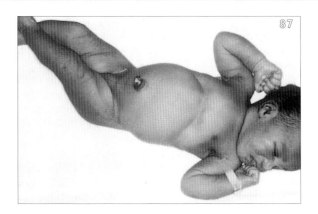

87 This male infant has been diagnosed with BPD and is demonstrating respiratory distress (87).
i. What are the signs of distress evident in this child, and what are other signs of distress that might be seen?
ii. What do you know about developmental delays and the child with BPD? Is this child at any risk?
iii. The nurse caring for this child can design the care provided to minimize stress and energy expenditure. What are some elements of this care?

88 An eight-month-old male infant has been brought to the Emergency Department by ambulance. The mother reports that he had stopped breathing, but was fine by the time the ambulance arrived. The paramedics report that the infant was a little distressed, but breathing and fully conscious.

The boy has been admitted to the children's wards several times with varying symptoms, including fits, cyanosis, vomiting, and respiratory arrest. In the past he has had a range of investigations including EEG and EKG (ECG), but no abnormalities have been identified. The nursing staff have never witnessed any fits or cyanotic episodes.

The child was born at 41 weeks' gestation and admitted at the age of three weeks with an URI and vomiting. His father works away from home, frequently absent for weeks at a time. His mother worked as a nursery nurse on a Special Care Baby Unit in a local hospital. She admits to being quite lonely, and not having friends in her own neighborhood.
i. Bearing in mind the past history of this child, what agencies should be working together to assess the child's needs?
ii. What is the role of the nurse in these situations?

87 i. The child shows evidence of grunting, flaring, retractions, tachypnea and abdominal respirations; he probably also has decreased feeding tolerance, wheezing, tachycardia, changes in oxygen saturation, color changes, anxiety, and irritability characteristic of BPD.

ii. The child with BPD is at very high risk of neurodevelopmental delays. Motor sequelae, including hypotonia, hypertonia, and delayed motor development, are frequently seen in the first year of life. The presence of IVH, PVL, or echodensity in the newborn period are all predictors for poor developmental outcome. Regular and recurring assessment and therapy with early intervention are essential.

iii. The nurse should try to eliminate noise, laughter, radios in patient areas; cluster care (grouping nursing activities together to maximize rest periods to the extent possible); provide positional supports such as blanket rolls and swaddling; become attuned to signs and symptoms of infant stress such as finger splay, hyperalert stare, color changes, hiccoughs, sneezes, frantic body movements, gaze aversion, and changes in vital signs.

88 i. In the UK, a consultant pediatrician (in the US, the attending physician) must be the lead officer in this child's case, particularly as induced illness such as Münchausen syndrome by proxy is now suspected. Clear hospital guidelines should dictate a course of action, which will not prejudice the child's safety.

A meeting of health professionals including the family doctor and health visitor (public health nurse) should be arranged as a matter of urgency. The purpose of this would be to share information about all the health problems and attendances at the Emergency Department, family doctor's clinic, or child health clinic. An assessment of the mother's health should also be made.

Monitoring of the mother and child is of the utmost importance and the other agencies can assist with this process.

At this stage the mother will not be involved in the decision-making process, to ensure the child's safety.

ii. The nurse should ensure that she maintains a comprehensive set of notes about the care of the child, types of investigations undertaken, and the relationship of the child/mother. All staff must maintain a nonjudgemental attitude.

The nurse will be expected to attend case conferences arranged with the other agencies to determine how the child's safety and welfare can be maintained.

89 A seven-year-old male developed lymphadenopathy, hepatomegaly, and spleno-megaly and was critically ill when first diagnosed with acute lymphoblastic leukemia. It is important to remember that most children presenting with this condition will not show such a degree of disease involvement and may only be visually pale.

i. What clinical signs may a child have when presenting with this condition?

ii. What implications to nursing care may anemia, thrombocytopenia, and neutro-penia have?

iii. What treatments may a child diagnosed with leukemia receive?

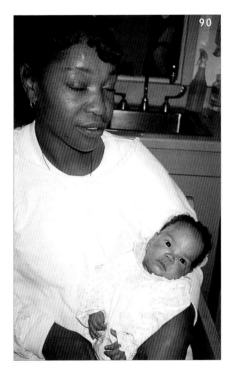

90 This eight-month-old male (90) was born to a 32-year-old mother who drank alcohol throughout her pregnancy. As a result he has FAS.

i. What amount of alcohol consumption causes FAS?

ii. What facial features are suggestive of FAS?

iii. What long-term behavioral concerns exist for infants and children with FAS?

89 i. Leukemia is a primary disorder of the bone marrow in which the normal marrow elements are replaced by immature or undifferentiated lymphocyte cells called blast cells. When the quantity of normal cells is depleted the marrow is unable to maintain peripheral blood elements within normal ranges, leading to anemia, thrombocytopenia, and neutropenia. Leukemia cells can be found anywhere within the body; however, they have an affinity for lymphoid tissue and can predominantly cause hepatomegaly, splenomegaly, and lymph gland enlargement.

ii. Throughout initial diagnosis and treatment these may occur at differing degrees for individual patients. Nursing interventions support medical treatment and involve the education of the family, daily monitoring of blood levels, blood transfusions for anemia, and platelet transfusion for thrombocytopenia.

Antibiotic support may be required in periods of neutropenia to prevent septic episodes.

Monitoring and correction of any of the above enables the family to spend as much time as possible at home.

iii. Treatment regimens follow strict protocols throughout the world. Treatments vary depending on diagnosis and stage of disease. The main treatment will follow a course of chemotherapy. Those patients who also present with central nervous system disease will also receive cranial irradiation.

Patients in high-risk groups, such as those with chromosomal translocations and those who relapse, will be offered bone marrow transplantation following initial treatment.

90 i. FAS has been associated with both small and large amounts of alcohol consumption, such that there is no definitive amount known to cause the condition.

ii. The characteristic facial features of FAS include microcephaly, a hypoplastic maxilla, micrognathia, a short nose, a smooth philtrum, and short palpebral fissures. Occasionally eyelid ptosis and epicanthic folds are seen.

iii. Infants with FAS frequently demonstrate irritability, tremulousness, hypotonia, motor retardation, and hearing disorders. Hyperactivity develops in childhood. Some degree of mental retardation or learning difficulty is present in approximately 80% of children with FAS.

91 A male toddler with a cervical liga-
mentous injury was admitted after a
motor vehicle collision (**91**). He was
appropriately restrained a child safety
seat when the car, which was traveling at
about 50 mph (80 kph), hit a wall. He
arrived in the Emergency Department
immobilized in his seat.

i. How do you assess for cervical spine injury in the toddler?

ii. What interventions and X-ray studies
should you prepare the patient and family
for?

iii. What discharge recommendations do
you give to the family?

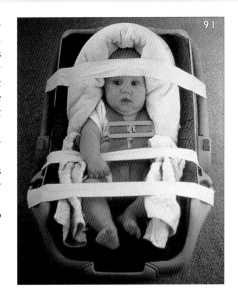

Urea 10.0 mmol/l (BUN 60.0 mg/dl)
K^+ 7.0 mmol/l (mEq/l)
Albumin 35.0 g/l (3.5 g/dl)

92 A 15-year-old male arrives at the
dialysis unit to receive his renal replacement therapy. His predialysis laboratory
values are shown above.

i. What type of dialysis machine is pictured (**92**), and what does it do?

ii. What laboratory value would be of
greatest concern, and why?

iii. What changes can be observed that are
associated with the abnormal value?

  The urea level drops from 10.0 mmol/l
(BUN 60.0 mg/dl) predialysis to a level of
2.5 mmol/l (BUN 15.0 mg/dl) postdialysis.

iv. What would you expect the albumin
level to be postdialysis, and why?

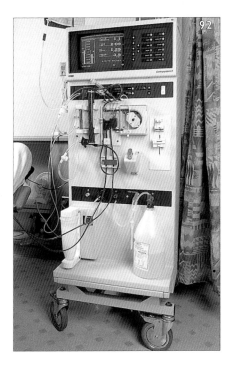

91 i. Developmentally, toddlers are unable to clearly identify sensation correctly and therefore it may be difficult to localize injuries. After a cursory primary survey, the child should be removed from the car seat while maintaining cervical and full body immobilization, then restrained supine on a backboard. The secondary survey will include a full neurologic and musculoskeletal assessment. If pain is noted on palpation of the neck, or active and passive motion are limited, radiographic evaluation is indicated.

ii. Initially, lateral and anterior–posterior cervical spine radiographs are done to determine if there are vertebral body fractures or subluxation. The entire cervical spine must be visualized from C1 through C7, including the top of T1, for the radiologist to determine if the cervical spine is radiographically negative. An open-mouth odontoid view of C1–C2 is usually not helpful in children aged under five years because ossification has not occurred. Active flexion and extension radiographs of the cervical spine are done if the child is able to follow commands. In the toddler and infant, an experienced clinician should apply gentle flexion and extension for the procedure. A CT and MRI may be necessary if the clinical examination and radiographic findings are inconclusive or inconsistent.

iii. Family discharge teaching should include signs and symptoms of neck injury including the inability to hold the head up and in neutral position, change in activity level, and loss of milestones such as not sitting, standing, or holding objects in the hands. The family should be instructed to contact their pediatrician or nurse practitioner immediately if changes or concerns develop. The car seat should be examined for structural damage and replaced if any cracks or dents appear in the frame or moldings, or if the straps were cut during extrication.

92 i. A hemodialysis machine. The machine filters the blood to remove wastes and excess electrolytes from the body.

ii. The potassium elevation would be the most problematic. The concern would be that when K^+ levels reach ≥ 7.0 mmol/l (mEq/l), alterations in the EKG (ECG) are seen.

iii. When the K^+ level is elevated, the EKG waves are altered, changing the T waves so that they look tented.

iv. Postdialysis, the albumin level should remain the same as it was predialysis, namely 35.0 g/l (3.5 g/dl). The reason that the value would remain unchanged is that the protein is not removed with this method of dialysis.

93 This five-month-old, ex-25 week premature female infant (93) had a Grade III IVH in the first week of life. As a result, she developed hydrocephalus and required a ventriculoperitoneal shunt.

i. How does a ventriculoperitoneal shunt treat hydrocephalus?

ii. What are the most common complications of ventriculoperitoneal shunts?

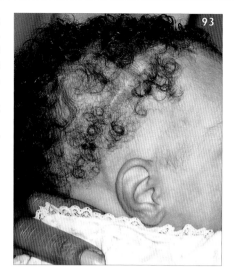

94 A 13-year-old female is playing soccer and falls directly on her left elbow. She has immediate pain and inability to move her left arm. She is splinted and brought to the local Emergency Department. X-rays are taken. She is diagnosed with a left elbow dislocation and radial head fracture.

i. After viewing the X-ray (94), describe the three most serious complications that can result from this injury.

Upon initial assessment, the patient complains of painful tingling in the fourth and fifth digits of the left hand. She exhibits profound sensory deficits in both fingers. She is unable to flex either digit. She cannot abduct or adduct the fingers. The thumb, index, and middle fingers have less than 5 mm (0.2 in) two-point discrimination. All five digits are warm and pink and have capillary refill of <2 seconds. Her radial pulse is 2+.

ii. What is the most likely cause of the symptoms described?

iii. The patient is taken to surgery and undergoes an open reduction with internal fixation. Postoperatively, what are the priorities for the nurse taking care of this patient?

93 i. Hydrocephalus is a condition caused by an imbalance in the production and absorption of CSF in the ventricular system. When the production is greater than absorption, CSF accumulates, producing passive dilation of the ventricles. A ventriculoperitoneal shunt provides drainage of the CSF from the ventricles to the peritoneum. Most shunts consist of a ventricular catheter, unidirectional flow valve, and a distal catheter. The valves are designed to open at a predetermined intraventricular pressure and close when the pressure falls below a predetermined level.

ii. The most common complications of ventriculoperitoneal shunts are infection and malfunction. Shunt infection is the most serious complication. It is more likely to occur in the one to two months following shunt placement but can occur at any time. A persistent infection of the shunt may require removal of the shunt and external drainage until the infection clears. Malfunctions include kinking, plugging, and separation or migration of the tubing. Shunt obstruction is often manifested by increased intracranial pressure. Surgical correction of the malfunction is necessary.

94 i. The three most serious complications to occur after a trauma of this nature are:

- Vascular injury.
- Nerve injury.
- Compartment syndrome.

ii. The ulnar nerve arises from the seventh and eighth cervical and first thoracic nerves. It descends down the arm past the elbow between the medial epicondyle and olecranon. It then passes across the forearm and wrist and into the fingers. The ulnar nerve is responsible for abduction and adduction of the fingers and sensation and flexion of the fourth and fifth digits. Severe trauma to the elbow can cause injury to the ulnar nerve.

iii. The priorities are:

- The nurse should monitor the patient's neurovascular status, with a focus on assessing for signs of compartment syndrome: excessive pain in the arm and on passive movement of fingers, pallor, absence of pulse, paralysis, and parathesia.
- Maintaining elevation of the left arm above the heart.
- Pain management using opioids initially, nonopioids after two to three days.

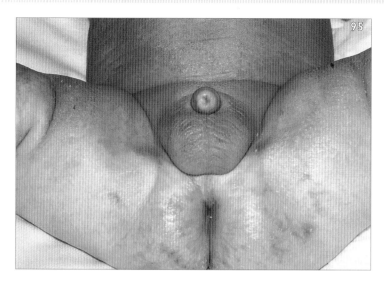

95 A one-month-old male infant develops an erythematous rash in his diaper (nappy) area (95). It is sharply demarcated and has numerous satellite lesions that extend beyond the larger lesion.

i. What type of rash does this infant have?

ii. What nursing measures will improve both the infant's condition and comfort?

	Breakfast	**Lunch**	**Dinner**	**Bedtime**
Monday	12.75 (237)	6.10 (113)	5.49 (102)	7.50 (140)
Tuesday	16.40 (305)	7.00 (130)	5.51 (103)	7.75 (144)
Wednesday	14.15 (363)	6.10 (113)	7.00 (130)	6.45 (119)
Thursday	17.20 (320)	6.40 (119)	6.65 (124)	6.70 (124)
Friday	14.70 (273)			

96 A five and a half-year-old female with a nine-month history of type 1 diabetes mellitus has the above blood glucose pattern (concentrations in mmol/l (mg/dl)).

i. What are possible explanations for the pattern of fasting hyperglycemia?

ii. What additional information needs to be collected in order to identify the source of the problem and recommend the appropriate intervention?

iii. Given this child's short history of diabetes mellitus, how could you explain this to her parents?

95 & 96: Answers

95 i. This infant has a *Candida* diaper dermatitis. The warm, moist atmosphere created in the diaper area provides an optimal environment for candidal growth.

ii. An anticandidal ointment is applied to the affected area four times per day until the rash clears. The diaper area should be kept as clean and dry as possible. Diapers should be changed as soon as they are wet or soiled. The diaper area should be exposed to air several times per day to facilitate drying. Barrier ointments, such as petroleum jelly, can be placed over the anticandidal ointment to aid in the healing of open lesions.

96 i. There are three possible reasons for fasting hyperglycemia. (1) Not enough insulin in the evening. (2) Too much insulin in the evening. (3) An appropriate amount of evening insulin, but its duration of action is not sufficiently long to carry over to the next morning.

ii. It is important to carry out further assessment in order to distinguish which of the above is the causative factor, as all three possibilities have very different interventions:

- First, collect more data. For several nights in a row, the girl needs to test her blood glucose around 00:00–04:00, or 6–8 hours after the evening insulin dose is given.
- If the middle of the night blood glucose is high (generally >10.2 mmol/l (>190 mg/dl)), more insulin is needed. Increasing the intermediate-acting insulin in the evening will help to prevent this hyperglycemia.
- Low 02:00–04:00 blood glucose (<3.2 mmol/l (<60 mg/dl)) will stimulate a release of counter-regulatory hormones in response to the insulin-induced hypoglycemia. When hypoglycemia precedes hyperglycemia, it is known as the 'Somogyi phenomenon'. Lowering the evening intermediate-acting insulin by 10–15% will prevent the hypoglycemia which triggers the rebound hyperglycemia.
- If the 00:00–04:00 glucose is normal (4.3–8.6 mmol/l (80–160 mg/dl)) and much higher than this by breakfast, this reflects the waning effects of biologically available insulin. This pattern is called the 'dawn phenomenon'. Moving the evening intermediate insulin to bedtime may delay its peak of action enough to coincide with this early morning pattern of hyperglycemia. The short-acting insulin should remain injected prior to the evening meal.

iii. This child may be leaving the 'honeymoon phase' of her diabetes mellitus. Honeymoon occurs for a short time after the onset and can last a few weeks to several months. During this time, there is endogenous insulin production from residual islet cells in the pancreas, and the child will require much less exogenous insulin during this time. The blood glucose pattern above may be reflective of too much exogenous insulin, leading to rebound hyperglycemia. The child's parents will need to keep in touch with the health-care team to receive help with lowering the dose. During this time, some children need only one injection of insulin per day. Most must continue to test the blood glucose regularly because eventually the residual islet cells will be destroyed by the same autoimmune process that caused the diabetes mellitus initially. A gradual increase in the average blood glucose signals the end of the 'honeymoon' and, likewise, the need for increased exogenous insulin.

97 A 15-year-old male was diagnosed with osteogenic sarcoma one month ago. He has completed three courses of chemotherapy and has just been scheduled for an above-the-knee amputation. The orthopedic surgeon tells the adolescent he will have a prosthesis after surgery.

i. Would you expect the adolescent to have pain after surgery, and for how long might this last?

ii. When should his parents expect that he would be able to be out of bed and begin ambulating?

iii. What signs of infection should the adolescent and his parents look for when he is discharged?

iv. By referring to the figure (97), describe to the parents and adolescent what the prosthesis will look like.

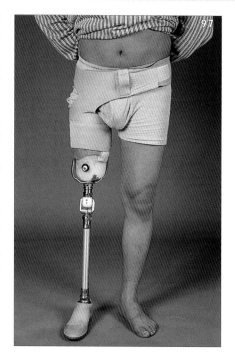

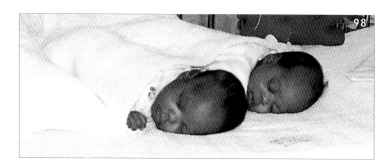

98 Co-bedding of twins in the neonatal ICU offers some physiologic or psychosocial benefits for newborns who may eventually share beds when discharged home. These infants (98) spend many hours together in the hospital in their co-bedding environment.

i. What are the potential benefits and potential risks to this practice?

ii. What recommendations should be made if co-bedding is done in the neonatal ICU?

97 & 98: Answers

97 i. The patient will experience two types of pain following surgery: postoperative incisional pain and phantom limb pain. Post-operative incisional pain is managed with opioids for a few days to two weeks. Phantom limb pain occurs later and is managed with TENS, neuropathic pain medications (carbamazepine (Tegretol) or gabapentin (Neurontin)), or ancillary pain medications (amitriptyline (Elavil)) or a combination of these.

ii. The patient should expect to be out of bed within 48–72 hours of surgery to prevent postoperative pneumonia. Postoperative orthopedic teaching will also include range of motion of the affected limb to prevent contractures (this involves sitting and lying on the abdomen), ambulating with crutches, and wrapping the stump to begin shaping for prosthesis fitting.

iii. Redness, swelling, drainage, an unusual smell at the incision site, or fever.

iv. The prosthesis consists of a plastic-type 'bucket' into which the pelvis 'sits' and is secured by a Velcro belt. This is attached to a metal, jointed appliance which includes a foot.

98 i. Many possible benefits include increased bonding and easier transition to home; continuing the developmental relationship that existed *in utero* with the sibling close by; lessening of the stressful environments through supportive mutual relationships between siblings. Potential risks include the higher chance for errors related to caring for the different infants. There is also a chance of increased exposure to problems, such as infections or even therapies such as oxygen, from one infant to the other.

ii. Both infants should be stable. Both twins should be clearly 'labeled' so that monitors or treatments are matched appropriately. Both twins should be paired in one nurse assignment. Both twins should be free from signs or symptoms of infection. At all times, a second isolate should be immediately available and warmed should the twins need to be separated for any reason.

WBC	$4 \times 10^9/l$ ($\times 10^3/\mu l$)
Hemoglobin	90 g/l (9 g/dl)
Hematocrit	0.27 l/l (27%)
Platelets	$110 \times 10^9/l$ ($\times 10^3/\mu l$)
Segmented neutrophils	$10 \times 10^9/l$ ($\times 10^3/\mu l$)
Lymphocytes	$43 \times 10^9/l$ ($\times 10^3/\mu l$)
Monocytes	$35 \times 10^9/l$ ($\times 10^3/\mu l$)
Band neutrophils	$2 \times 10^9/l$ ($\times 10^3/\mu l$)

99 A routine weekly CBC for an eight-month-old infant with HIV disease yields the results shown above.
i. What is an ANC, and how is it calculated?
ii. What is this infant's ANC?
iii. What nursing measures should be instituted for this ANC?

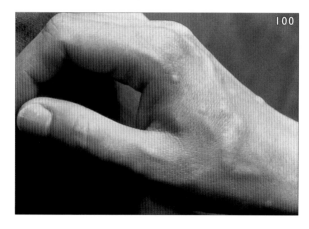

100 A 12-year-old male with myelomeningocele arrives for a routine clinic visit. The mother states that, during the drive to the clinic, her child was playing with a balloon that was given to him at a local restaurant. The child had an obvious urticarial rash on his hand (**100**).
i. What is the probable etiology of this urticarial reaction?
ii. What are four potential routes for latex exposure?
iii. What latex sensitivity precautions should this child take?
iv. At what point should latex precautions be initiated on a child with spina bifida?

99 i. ANC is a calculation performed by using the patient's CBC to determine their ability to handle bacterial infections:

ANC = % neutrophils × WBC
% neutrophils = (segmented neutrophils + band neutrophils) × 10

ii.   ANC = (segmented neutrophils + band neutrophils) × WBC × 10
ANC = (10 + 2) × 4 × 10
ANC = 480

iii. An ANC of <1,000 suggests that the patient is at greater risk of bacterial infections. Thorough handwashing, appropriate room selection in a noninfectious area, restricting visitors and hospital personnel with active infection, and maintaining adequate nutrition and rest are appropriate nursing interventions to protect the patient with a low ANC.

100 i. A latex sensitivity reaction from touching the rubber balloon.
ii. Four potential routes of latex exposure are:

- Inhalation (breathing in airborne powder from latex gloves or deflating latex balloons).
- Ingestion (eating food that has been handled by workers wearing latex gloves).
- Intravenous (injecting medicine through latex ports).
- Direct contact.

iii. The child should take several precautions to prevent himself from being exposed to latex. He should avoid contact with all products containing latex. In case exposure does occur, an antihistamine should be kept in the home to treat mild skin reactions. All individuals having contact with the child such as dentists, primary care physicians, day-care workers, therapists, and school officials should be informed of the child's latex sensitivity and the need for precautions to be taken. In addition, a medical alert bracelet or necklace, that identifies the child as having a latex sensitivity, should be worn by the affected child.
iv. All children with myelomeningocele should be treated as latex-sensitive from birth. Minimizing exposure early in life may limit the occurrence or severity of sensitivity reactions.

101 A 12-month-old male presents to the Emergency Department with acute onset of seizures and coma. The parents describe that, over the past week, this previously healthy child has been more sleepy than usual, is no longer able to walk (he started walking at 10 months), had a decreased appetite, and occasional vomiting. The only recent change related to the child's feedings is that the mother reports using a new method of boiling water to prepare the formula. On presentation the child is afebrile with normal vital signs. The hematocrit is 0.314 l/l (31.4%) and the electrolytes are normal. A toxic screen is sent which is normal. A lead screen reveals 3.75 µmol/l (78 µg/dl).

i. What is the diagnosis?

ii. What are the symptoms usually associated with this diagnosis?

iii. What are the common sources of this toxic agent?

iv. What prevention strategies will you discuss with the parents to prevent this?

102 A four-year-old female with cystic fibrosis is admitted to the hospital with a one-week history of increased cough, difficulty breathing, and dyspnea. Her fevers reached a maximum of 39°C (102.2°F), and her sputum is green and thick. Sputum culture and sensitivity results are shown. The child is pale, her O$_2$ saturation is 90%. Clubbing is 3+ (**102**). Her body weight is 13.8 kg (30 lb 6 oz), down from 14 kg (30 lb 13 oz) two weeks ago. She is started on an aggressive course of chest physiotherapy after nebulizer therapy (salbuterol [salbutamol; Albuterol] 0.5 ml with 2 ml normal saline) t.i.d.

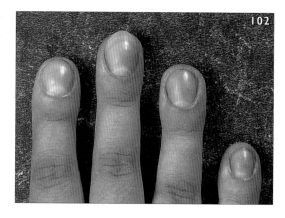

Moderate mixed oropharyngeal flora
Moderate nonmucoid *Pseudomonas aeruginosa*
Moderate mucoid *Pseudomonas aeruginosa*

i. What nursing strategies can be utilized to enhance this child's cooperation with therapies?

ii. Based on the sputum culture results, which treatment modalities would be most appropriate to meet her needs during this acute exacerbation?

iii. What symptoms of further deterioration should be looked for?

101 & 102: Answers

101 i. Acute lead encephalopathy.

ii. Acute symptoms of lead poisoning in children, (coma, seizures, lethargy, anorexia, vomiting, abdominal pain, loss of recently acquired skill) are rarely noted until the serum lead level is >2.5 μmol/l (>52 μg/dl). Chronic symptoms, associated with levels <2.5 μmol/l (<52 μg/dl), should be screened for. These include detailed environmental history, developmental screening, family history of lead poisoning, history of pica, and laboratory measurements including lead level, hematocrit, hemoglobin, iron, and erythrocyte protoporphyrin.

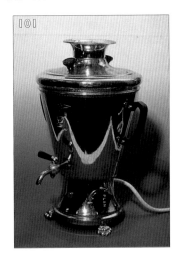

Serum lead levels as low as 0.5 μmol/l (10.3 μg/dl) have been associated with harmful effects, such as developmental delay; therefore, it is important both to screen children for lead and educate parents about sources of lead.

iii. The most common source of lead poisoning is lead-based paint. Poisoning occurs when the child ingests the chipped or peeling paint or paint-contaminated soil, dust, or water. Additional, although rare, sources of lead include lead solder found in old pipes or containers. The urn illustrated (**101**) was used to heat water for the child in the present case. Further investigation revealed lead solder used to weld all joints in the urn.

iv. Parents should be educated about the environmental sources of lead. Caution should be taken in homes with lead-based paint. Cleaning of lead paint surfaces, floors, and window sills with a phosphate-based cleaner twice weekly can reduce the risk of contamination. However, abatement of lead-based paint from the home, by a trained expert, is essential for permanent removal of the risk. Any container used for cooking of food, eating, and heating of liquids should be free of lead-based solder.

102 i. Pre-school children with a chronic illness are developing autonomy and have a need for control over their environment. Alternate the child's aerosol treatments and chest physiotherapy with time for play. Reward her for cooperation with the treatment plan. Utilization of dolls and therapeutic play may decrease her anxiety.

ii. The primary treatment modalities are antibiotics, either aerosolized or intravenous, aggressive nutrition, and intensive chest therapy. Antibiotics are given usually over two weeks, most often very high doses of aminoglycosides. Two antibiotics are given concurrently to potentiate their effectiveness and decrease the development of antibiotic resistance.

iii. *Pseudomonas* infection, once acquired, can never be fully eliminated. Symptoms of worsening lung function can include increased fatigue, dyspnea, cyanosis, hemoptysis, and changes in color or consistency of sputum.

103 This X-ray (**103**) shows a child with radiopaque fluid flowing up from the bladder to the ureter.
i. What is the condition called, and what can be the consequences to the child?
ii. How can VUR be detected and managed? How can the pediatric nurse help the child?

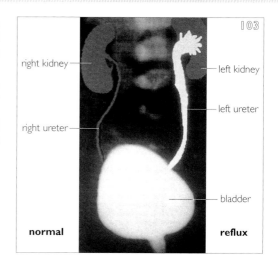

right kidney — — left kidney

— left ureter

right ureter —

— bladder

normal   **reflux**

104 An 18-month-old Caucasian female comes in for a well child examination. Her mother stays at home with her and is the primary caretaker. This child has had three DPT/HIB immunizations, three doses of OPV, and three hepatitis B immunizations. She missed her MMR at 15 months because she was febrile and was treated for a left otitis media infection. Today, her examination reveals an outgoing, verbal toddler who is healthy. Height and weight are age-appropriate. She is given an MMR #1 and DPT/HIB #4. Eleven days later, her mother calls to report that the child has

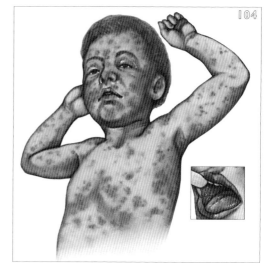

the measles and is covered with a red, raised rash from head to toe (**104**), but is not febrile. She is playful and her appetite is normal.
i. What is the likely cause of the rash?
ii. Should a child with such a rash be excluded from day-care or group activities?

103 i. The retrograde flow of urine from the bladder into one or both ureters is called VUR. It is usually congenital in origin, although it occasionally occurs following surgery, trauma, infection, or neoplastic involvement. VUR is asymptomatic and unless complicated by UTI is of no significance to the child. It is, however, found in 35% of children who are investigated by cystogram, following a proven UTI. Although the peak age incidence for the first attack of UTI is in the preschool years, there may be many young children whose VUR is never discovered because their UTI may go undetected.

In the presence of VUR and UTI, organisms can travel up the ureter(s) into the kidney(s) and induce scarring of the kidney tissue or RN. Although RN usually develops in early life its consequences, e.g., hypertension and loss of renal function, may not occur until many years later. RN accounts for 20% of all renal transplants performed in the UK annually.

ii. The only reliable way of detecting VUR is to perform a micturating cystogram, an invasive X-ray requiring the introduction of a catheter into the urethra. The nurse can help by ensuring the child and parents have time to understand the purpose of the investigation and the procedures to be used. Some children may be helped by play therapy using pictures, stories and/or a doll to familiarize themselves with the planned catheterization and X-ray.

VUR may be treated surgically or conservatively. Surgery involves reimplantation of the ureters into a new position in the bladder wall. However, conservative management is now usually preferred at least as a first option.

Management usually entails urinary surveillance to ensure prompt detection and treatment of UTI and sometimes the administration of prophylactic antibiotics in an effort to prevent the development of UTI. The aim of this strategy is to prevent or minimize the development of new or exacerbation of existing RN.

The nurse can assist the family by advising on the appropriate method for urine collection, ensuring that an adequate supply of urine-collecting equipment is available. Secondly, by educating parents to recognize signs and symptoms of possible UTIs, e.g. unexplained fever, being generally unwell for no specific reason.

104 i. Given that this rash occurred within two weeks of receiving an MMR vaccine, the first suspicion should be a reaction to the MMR vaccine. About 5% of children vaccinated will break out in a measles-like rash at 10–14 days after receiving the immunization. Approximately 5–15% of children receiving the vaccine will become febrile around the fifth or sixth day following an MMR vaccination. The fever usually lasts one or two days, but could last as long as five days. The rash and a fever usually do not occur together.

ii. Children with a vaccine-induced rash from an MMR vaccine are not considered contagious and do not need to be excluded from day-care or group activity.

105 A 16-year-old male is a passenger on a motorcycle when the vehicle is struck by a car. He sustains a grade I open fracture of the right tibia and fibula, the size of the open wound being <10 cm (<4 in). He is rushed to hospital and brought to surgery where he undergoes irrigation and débridement of the wound and an open reduction with internal fixation of the fracture. Four months later, the patient begins having drainage from the right tibial wound. Nine months later, X-rays indicate that there is no evidence of bone healing at the fracture site.

The physical examination reveals a large indurated area over the midshaft of his right tibia. Purulent drainage appears from a sinus tract. His neurovascular examination is normal. The patient complains of severe pain along the tibia. His ESR is 56 mm/hr.

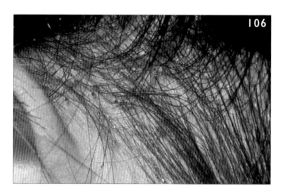

i. What is the patient's probable medical diagnosis?
ii. What is the significance of his ESR?
iii. When you prepare the adolescent and parents for surgery, what should you tell them about the surgical apparatus (105)?
iv. What complications can result from this procedure?
v. Before discharge, what should the nurse provide the patient with in terms of patient education?
vi. When will this patient be allowed to fully weight bear on his right leg?

106 This child (106) was sent to the school nurse by her teacher with persistent hair scratching.
i. What suspicions should a nurse have immediately when a child is described like this?
ii. What advice should the nurse give to the child's parents?
iii.. What advice should the nurse give to the child's teacher?

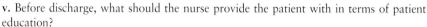

105 i. This patient has an unhealed bone with signs of osteomyelitis: purulent drainage, pain, induration, and an elevated ESR. This problem is also known as an infected nonunion. Osteomyelitis will prevent healing in a fractured bone.

ii. The ESR is an indication of an infectious process.

iii. The apparatus is called the Ilizarov External Fixator. When the patient is taken to surgery, the hardware is removed with copious irrigation to the bone. The diseased portion of the bone is resected and a circular fixator applied. The patient will undergo a process called bone transport which will regenerate and restore the resected segment.

iv. Complications that can result from this procedure include: infection, nerve injury, injury to a vascular structure, knee and ankle contractures, and nonunion of the newly formed bone. The most common complication encountered by these patients is pin site infections.

v. Pre-discharge education will include:

• Pin care.
• Signs and symptoms of infection.
• Neurovascular checks.
• Range of motion exercises.

The patient will be taught to turn the nuts attached to the long telescoping rods using 10-mm wrenches. He will be instructed to turn each of the four nuts one-quarter of a turn, four times a day. This process is known as 'distraction', which is the mechanical separation of two opposing bone ends. By turning the nuts one-quarter of a turn four times a day, the patient will transport a fragment of bone across the gap 1 mm per day. As this intercalary fragment moves across this space it will leave a fibrous trail of bone behind it. Eventually, this will ossify and the gap will be replaced by healthy new bone. The patient begins distractions after a latency period of three to seven days after surgery

vi. Because of the stability of this fixator, the patient is allowed to fully weight bear in the immediate postoperative period. Later, as osteogenesis takes place, full weight bearing will encourage faster healing of the bone.

106 i. With the description of a child who is persistent with head scratching, the school nurse should immediately assess the child for pediculosis. Although the head lice may not always be visible in different colors or textures of hair, the scalp spots that result from bites are a good indication to inspect closely. Nits can be seen on hair shafts.

ii. Head lice must be treated and the parents can assume that the family has also been infected. All members of the family should wash their hair with an insecticidal shampoo, as well as washing their bed covers, hats, or other articles of clothing that can facilitate the spread of head lice to others. (See also **40.**)

iii. Pediculosis is extremely contagious. All children should be screened. Notes should be sent home to the parents alerting them of head lice cases at school.

107 A two-year-old female was referred to an otolaryngologist after experiencing six episodes of otitis media in an eight-month period. It is reported that she has had persistent bilateral effusions for the past six months. A bilateral myringotomy and tube placement was recommended. The child otherwise has no prior medical history. Her parents report that she has achieved all of her developmental milestones; however, her vocabulary at this time consists of approximately 10 single words. The parents are also concerned about what they could have done to help prevent the multiple occurrences of her ear infections.

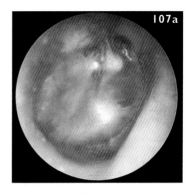

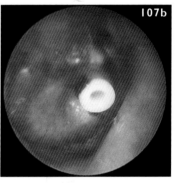

i. What otoscopic signs differentiate chronic from acute otitis (107a)?
ii. What population is at greater risk of recurrent/chronic otitis media with effusion?
iii. What are the risk factors associated with otitis media?
iv. What is the purpose of the tympanotomy tubes? What teaching should be done with the parents after PE tubes are inserted (107b)?

108 A 14-year-old Hispanic male presents to the Emergency Department with dyspnea, chest tightness, cough, a pulse oximetry reading of 90%, and a PEFR which is 40% of normal. His PEFR has been steadily decreasing over the past three days since he visited his grandmother's farm. He has a known allergy to dogs and cats. He is on a steroid inhaler (beclomethasone, two puffs b.i.d.), with a beta-agonist inhaler (salbuterol [salbutamol; Albuterol], two puffs q.i.d.) p.r.n. He is treated every 30 minutes × 2 with salbuterol 1 ml in 2 ml of normal saline via a nebulizer. His pulse oximetry values increase to 98%, PEFR to 85%, the chest tightness and dyspnea are relieved, and his cough has decreased. He is sent home on salbuterol by MDI at two puffs q.i.d. with holding chamber until the cough has subsided, beclomethasone MDI four puffs t.i.d. × one week, four puffs b.i.d × one week, and then two puffs b.i.d. × one week, which was the maintenance dose for the child. He is also given 40 mg of oral prednisone for 5 days, and is told to return to the clinic in one week unless his symptoms return or his PEFR falls below 70% of normal.
i. What are the essential components of an office spirometry, and what does it tell us about asthma?
ii. Once the acute exacerbation has been stabilized, what important pharmacologic consideration was made?

107 i. The tympanic membrane is usually opaque, it can be retracted onto the ossicles, hypervascularization may be present, distortion of landmarks, and immobile tympanic membrane.

ii. High-risk populations include any child with:

- A facial–cranial abnormality.
- Down syndrome.
- Hearing impairment.
- There also tends to be a higher incidence in males.
- A history of otitis media in parent/siblings.
- Allergies.

iii. Environmental risk factors include:

- Day-care centers.
- Smoking in the home.
- Seasonal, with greater occurrences in the autumn/winter months.
- Siblings in the home.
- Allergies.
- The role of the type of infant feeding (breast versus bottle) remains controversial.

iv. The main reason for the recurrence of ear infections is due to the dysfunction of the Eustachian tube, providing poor ventilation of the middle ear space. The purpose of the ventilation tubes is to aerate the middle ear space, to decrease accumulation of the fluid behind the tympanic membrane, and to reduce the occurrence, usually, of otitis media. Ear infections can continue to occur despite ventilation-type placement, but are significantly decreased. If an ear infection does develop, drainage will be seen from the affected ear(s). This signifies that the ventilation tubes are functioning and are allowing the infection to drain from the middle ear space. The drainage may be of mucus type, being white, yellow, green, or blood-tinged in nature. In this event, the patient is instructed to be evaluated and treated appropriately. Ventilation tubes stay in place on an average of 9–18 months. They gradually extrude themselves from the eardrum spontaneously. Most otolaryngologists recommend water precautions. Contamination of water into the middle ear space predisposes a child to otitis media. Water precautions have only to be observed until the tubes have extruded and confirmation that the insertion site has healed.

108 i. Spirometry typically measures the FVC, FEV_1, and FEF_{25-75}. The FEV_1 is the most specific and dependable measure of airway obstruction, the normal being 80–100% of predicted. It is believed that the FEF_{25-75} measures the obstruction in peripheral airways, and the normal is at least 50–60% of predicted. The reversibility with bronchodilators indicates asthma.

ii. In many asthma episodes there is an early and late response phase. The early phase is caused by bronchoconstriction and responds well to a bronchodilator. The late phase (after six to eight hours) is associated with increased airway reactivity and inflammation. Inhaled corticosteroids help to block the late phase. The oral steroids were given to decrease the inflammation that has built up over time and led to the onset of the exacerbation.

Zone	PEFR (l/min)	Action
Green	416–520	No asthma symptoms present. Take control medication as usual (beclomethasone, two puffs, b.i.d.)
Yellow	260–416	Take salbuterol (salbutamol; Albuterol), two puffs immediately. Asthma may not be under control. Consult a physician regarding increase in steroid medication or addition of a long-acting bronchodilator
Red	Below 260	**Medical alert.** Take short-acting bronchodilator immediately. Recheck PEFR in 20 minutes. If still in red zone, repeat bronchodilator and call the physician for further instruction. If it returns to the yellow or green zone, notify the physician for follow-up care

109 With regard to the patient in **108**, looking at the chart above, what peak flow monitored asthma action plan would you put in place for this patient if his peak flow personal best at this visit was 390 l/min on Monday morning before school?

110 This previously healthy, seven-year-old female fell off a trampoline and sustained a displaced right distal femur fracture. She was placed in 90/90 skeletal traction for nine days (**110a**). A spica cast was then applied to provide immobilization and allow for healing of the bone fracture.
i. What is the purpose of 90/90 skeletal traction?
ii. What should be included in the nurse's assessment of the skeletal traction apparatus?
iii. What assessment and nursing interventions are required in caring for the pin site of a child in skeletal traction?

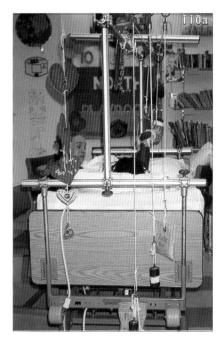

109 The yellow zone is where this patient is, and he would be told to take two puffs of salbuterol immediately and make an appointment with the clinic.

110 i. Skeletal traction applies traction directly to the bone through the use of pins, wires, or tongs. This hardware is inserted through the bone distal to the fracture site or deformity and is attached to traction weights through ropes and pulleys. Skeletal traction provides a continuous pull along the long axis of the bone and permits longer periods of immobilization than other forms of traction. Skeletal traction is applied to

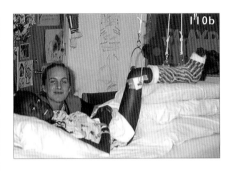

reduce or immobilize fractures until callus forms and calcification begins; to realign bone fragments; to reduce pain or muscle spasms; to expand joint spaces prior to surgery; and to provide rest to a diseased or injured body part. 90/90 traction is a treatment modality used for children with displaced fractures of the femur. A Steinmann pin or Kirschner wire is placed in the distal femur fragment of the femur with the child's lower leg in either a short leg cast or supported in a sling. This traction allows a 90° flexion of both the hip and the knee. The child must remain in 90/90 traction until satisfactory alignment and early healing is achieved as determined by serial X-rays.

ii. Caring for a child in traction involves the care and maintenance of the traction apparatus. The angles of the ropes and pulleys should create a pull along the axis of the bone (**110b**). This should be checked routinely, especially after changing the linens. Altering the line of pull can misalign the bone, resulting in muscle spasms, pain, displacement, or delayed healing. Ropes should be taut and run freely through the pulleys. Knots should be secure and ropes should be checked for fraying. The nurse should ensure that the amount of weight matches the physician's order and that the weights are hanging freely, clear of the bed and off the floor. Traction should be maintained continuously; therefore, the weights should not be lifted when moving the patient in bed.

iii. A pin site is vulnerable to infection because the hardware pierces the skin and enters the bone. An infection can easily spread to the bone causing osteomyelitis, a serious complication of skeletal traction. The pin sites should be assessed several times a day for signs of infection including edema, redness, localized warmth, and purulent drainage. Specific cleansing practices vary but the most commonly used solution is hydrogen peroxide. The pin site should be pressed firmly with a sterile cotton swab to help prevent scab formation and tenting of the skin around the pin. Following cleaning, a sterile 2 × 2 gauze with a slit may be applied or the pin may be left uncovered.

111 This child (**111a**) appears to be enjoying his ice-cream and companion but is likely to precipitate an acute problem. What can intervention in this situation prevent?

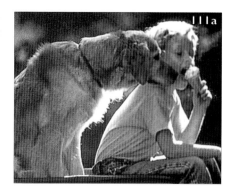

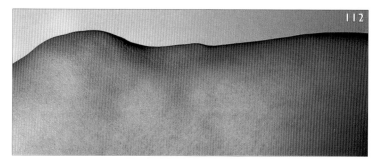

112 This young woman's unusually large tibial tuberosity (**112**) is suggestive of Osgood–Schlatter disease or osteochondrosis at the tibial physis.
i. From what past childhood experiences did this condition most likely result?
ii. What group of children are at risk of this condition, and what warnings should nurses give to them and their parents?

113 What are the most common 'trigger' factors that may precipitate an anaphylactic reaction?

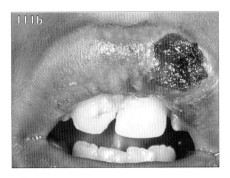 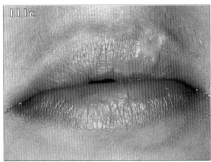

111 The lip photographed (**111b**) shows a deep puncture wound resulting from a dog competing for food with a child. The injury will likely result in a scar because of the location and extent of soft tissue damage (**111c**).

112 i. This condition may have been exacerbated by rigorous athletics during her adolescent years. Osgood–Schlatter disease occurs during periods of growth in long bones, when the cartilaginous physis (growth plate) may be particularly susceptible to trauma.
ii. The tibial tuberosity is the anatomical point of insertion for the quadriceps femoris. It is speculated by some that, due to the proximity of the insertion to the tibial physis, abnormally large muscular forces associated with sports or inappropriate physical training during adolescence may exacerbate this condition.

113 The most common 'trigger' factors that may precipitate an anaphylactic reaction are:

- Peanuts (common in children). Peanuts are not classed as true 'nuts', as they grow in the ground. They are related to the legume family – peas, beans, lentils. Children *do not* grow out of an allergy to peanuts – the allergy grows with them.
- True nuts, such as almonds, brazil nuts, walnuts, cashew, coconut.
- Fish and shell fish.
- Wasp and bee stings.
- Egg and dairy products.
- Natural latex.
- Penicillin or any other drug/injection.

114 Rotaviral diarrhea is generally a self-limiting disease and treatment is supportive, as no specific antiviral therapy is available. Dehydration and electrolyte abnormalities are the principle cause of serious morbidity.
i. What are the clinical differences in physical signs of varying degrees of dehydration?
ii. When is oral or intravenous fluid therapy preferable?

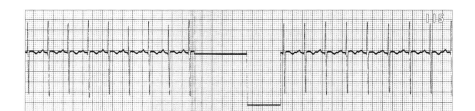

115 A mother and father bring in their five-year-old daughter, with symptoms of fever and malaise since her visit at the dentist. She has been a relatively healthy child who was born with tetralogy of Fallot and underwent surgical correction at one month of age. She is evaluated by her cardiologist every year. Her last visit was eight months ago. The EKG (ECG) rhythm (**115**) suggests possible problems that she may be experiencing.
i. What signs and symptoms would you evaluate to determine her present cardiac status? What EKG rhythms would suggest potential problems?
ii. What concerns do you have that her cardiac status has changed? What would be the appropriate intervention?
iii. What precautions for SBE should be discussed with her parents at every annual examination?

114 & 115: Answers

114 i. The clinical signs of dehydration range from mild to severe (see table).
ii. All acute diarrheal illnesses respond to fluid therapy, oral or intravenous. For the child who is mild to moderately dehydrated, oral fluid therapy is the preferred route to rehydrate rapidly, replace ongoing losses, and provide maintenance fluids. In the severely dehydrated child who is in shock or near shock, intravenous therapy is mandatory, as in any situation where oral therapy is impossible.

115 i. Physical signs of a child who has had cardiac repair include: growth failure, changes in perfusion, a new or changed heart murmur, tachycardia, bradycardia, arrhythmia, dyspnea, tachypnea, and/or a change in breath sounds. Symptoms that would be concerning include mood and behavior changes in the child. Her tachycardia from the EKG suggests further examination.
ii. A child with cardiac surgery with a fever and tachycardia will always concern you due to the

Degree	Symptoms
Mild	Slightly dry mucous membranes Alert Increased thirst Mild decreased urine output Tears present Elastic turgor Capillary refill <2 seconds Anterior fontanel and eyes normal Vital signs normal
Moderate	Lips and oral mucosa dry Irritable Moderately thirsty Urine output <1 ml/kg/hr Absent tears; tenting of skin Capillary refill 2–3 seconds Sunken anterior fontanel and eyes Heart/respiratory rate increased
Severe	Mucous membranes very dry Lethargic or comatose Oliguria Absent tears; cold, clammy skin Capillary refill >3 seconds Very sunken fontanel and eyes Heart/respiratory rate increased Blood pressure normal or reduced Weak pulse

potential for SBE. It would be appropriate to call her cardiologist to review your concerns. The cardiologist will work with you to determine what evaluations and/or treatments are required based on the magnitude of the problem.
iii. It is important to review the need for SBE prophylaxis with her parents at every annual examination. She will require SBE prophylaxis whenever she is to undergo a surgical procedure, including dental surgery. The recommendations for SBE prophylaxis are constantly evolving and changing, however, which makes her cardiologist the best resource for the most current recommendations.

116 A 42-year-old female is 10 weeks pregnant. This is her first pregnancy and she is concerned about having a child with Down syndrome.
i. Is there an increased risk for Down syndrome with advanced maternal age?
ii. When should prenatal screening and diagnostic testing be done?
iii. What is the nurse's role in prenatal diagnosis and genetic counseling?

117 This 25-week gestation former premature baby (**117**) was born with immature lungs resulting in chronic lung disease. Her medical complications from birth and her gastroesophageal reflux in the neonatal period has kept her hospitalized most of her life. What activities should be provided for long-term hospitalized children?

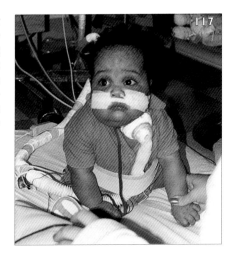

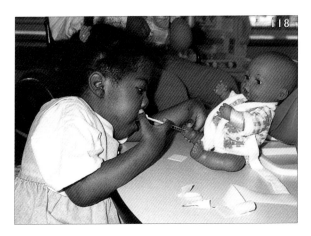

118 This preschool child (**118**) has been admitted for a club foot repair. What is she doing to the doll?

116 i. The graph (116) shows the increased incidence of Down syndrome with advanced maternal age.
ii. The most commonly used screening tests (see table) are the Triple Screen and alpha feto-protein plus, which are usually offered between 15–20 weeks gestation. Prenatal diagnosis of Down syndrome has an accuracy rate of 98–99%.
iii. The nurse's role in counseling women of advanced maternal age, or who have a family history of Down syndrome, should include a discussion of diagnostic testing. If the tests reveal a Down syndrome child, the nurse must encourage the parents to express their feelings concerning the pregnancy, elective abortion and support their decision to either continue or terminate the pregnancy.

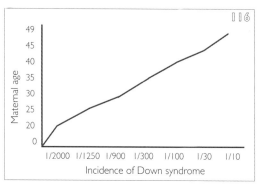

Screening test	Weeks of gestation
Chorionic villus sampling	8–12
Amniocentesis	12–20
Percutaneous umbilical blood sampling	After 20

117 Long-term hospitalization and therapies to treat infants' conditions compromise normal activities and contribute to the developmental problems that children have following chronic illnesses. Normal infancy is altered with hospital feedings, the noise of intensive care equipment, bright lights without day/night patterns, and frequent painful or unpleasant stimulation. Normal amounts and quality of stimulation should be a goal in the interventions planned. Exercise compatible with potential development and toys or interesting things to play with should be provided whenever possible. Providing a consistent caregiver can help the infant develop trust.

118 Children in the preschool period are cognitively and emotionally unprepared to be given preoperative instructions or preparation that are verbal alone. They need to experience information through play therapy and be provided with support to allow them to act out their misconceptions in a safe and pleasant manner. They can be assisted to understand what they will experience and they can be comforted by knowing that caregivers will be with them in the process. This child is engaging in play therapy. Preparation for surgery through play therapy can alleviate later anxieties and improve child cooperation. All of this can be enhanced with toys and the opportunity to handle medical supplies.

119 A 19-month-old male is brought to the clinic for a well child examination. His parents are farm workers who travel the country seeking seasonal work. There are three siblings in the household, ages four, seven, and nine years. An uncle living with the family has just been diagnosed with the AIDS virus. Height, weight, and head circumference are age-appropriate. Except for an ear infection four months ago, this child has been healthy. Antonio has had two DPT/HIB vaccines, two OPVs, and two hepatitis vaccines since birth.

i. Using the tables, identify which immunizations this child should receive at this visit. What common side-effects should the parents be told about?

ii. Which type of polio vaccine is indicated for this child, and why?

iii. When will Antonio be eligible for his fourth DPT/HIB vaccine?

iv. Are you concerned about the immunization status of the three siblings? If so, how could you intervene to determine if they are up to date?

US immunization schedule, birth to 6 years

Birth–2 months	Hepatitis B-1
1–4 months	Hepatitis B-2
2 months	DPT/HIB, polio
4 months	As above
6 months	DPT/HIB
6–18 months	Hepatitis B-3, polio
12–15 months	HIB, MMR
12–18 months	Varicella
15–18 months	DPT
4–6 years	DPT, polio, MMR

UK immunization schedule, birth to 5 years

2 months	Diptheria, whooping cough, tetanus, HIB, polio
3 months	As above
4 months	As above
12–18 months	MMR, HIB
3–5 years	DPT

120 This infant is receiving oxygen via a nasal cannula. (**120**) What are the principles of oxygen administration and specific practices related to nasal cannulas?

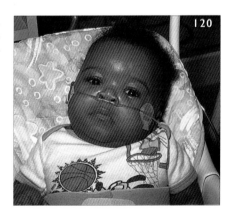

119 i. This is a transient family with a history of sporadic medical care. According to the recommendations in the US by the American Academy of Pediatrics, this child is in need of DPT/HIB #3, Polio #3, Hepatitis B #3 and MMR #1. These vaccines are compatible one with another. The probability that this child will return to your clinic for further care is very small. Therefore, all of the immunizations should be given at this visit. Every opportunity to immunize a well child should be taken, particularly one who is chronically behind or at high risk. Make sure that parents are given acetaminophen (paracetamol) to administer to minimize the child's discomfort. (Note: in the UK, these recommendations are slightly different.)
ii. IPV should be given to the child because of his uncle's recent diagnosis of AIDS. OPV is a live virus vaccine that is shed in the stool, saliva, and nasal secretions of the immunized child for six to eight weeks after vaccination. While this poses minimal threat to this toddler, an immunocompromised individual in the toddler's environment is at risk of infection. Since the uncle resides in the household and it is not feasible to isolate him for six to eight weeks, IPV is the best option. However, IPV is given by injection only and is more expensive than OPV.
iii. This toddler would be eligible for his next DPT/HIB #4 in six months. This should be clearly marked in the immunization record which has been updated and returned to his parents.
iv. Since this toddler is behind in his immunizations, it is probable that at least one of the other siblings is behind also. Ask the parents if they have immunization records for the other children with them. If they do, ask if you may review them. Write down any needed immunizations (make sure they are able to read before doing so) and give these to them before they leave. Offer to make an appointment for the other children before they leave the clinic and institute a referral to the public health or home visiting nurse.

120 Oxygen administration is specified per order including concentration and delivery method. Adequate humidity is necessary to prevent drying of the airways and can be delivered by jet nebulizer, cascade, bubbler, or other heated humidity systems. The duration of operation of the oxygen system will vary depending on the size of the tank, the flow rate in liters per minute, and the manufacturer. Nasal cannulas, although they can roll off easily during sleep, have distinct advantages for use during the waking hours of an infant without a tracheostomy. It offers the least restriction for the infant's visual, auditory, and motor environments. It should be held in place by a headband, tape, or a clear surgical adhesive dressing. If the cannula prongs do not fit the nares, they can be clipped off.

121 What are expected speech and language characteristics of a two-year-old child?

122 This three-year-old child (**122**) was a 25-week-old premature baby who has been on systemic steroids long term for chronic lung disease.
i. What characteristics or side-effects become possible in children on long-term steroids?
ii. What complications become critical in managing her care?

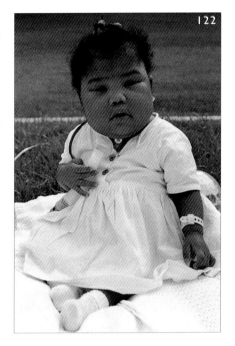

123 This 12-month-old female's gastrostomy site is red, swollen, tender, and warm (**123**). There is thick yellow drainage and ascending reddish streaks can be seen. The child has a low grade fever and is less active than usual.
i. What is the most likely clinical problem?
ii. What two factors predispose a child's gastrostomy site to become infected?
iii. What is the nurse's role in decreasing these factors?

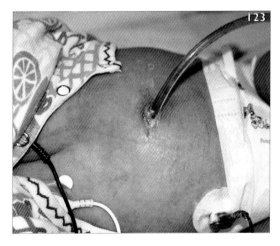

Age	Response
0–2 months	Coos, vocal sounds
2–6 months	Babbles
6–9 months	Babbles, uses repetition, e.g. lala, tata, dada
9–12 months	1–2 words, may still be unintelligible
12–18 months	4–50 words, develops jargon, 25% intelligible
18–24 months	50–200 words, two-word sentences, echolalia, 50% intelligible
2–2.5 years	200–300 words, two- to three-word sentences, 50% intelligible
2.5–3years	900 words, three-word sentences, 75% intelligible
3–4 years	900–1,500 words, four-word sentences, 100% intelligible
4–5 years	2,000 words, four- to five-word sentences, 100% intelligible
5–6 years	2,500+ words, five- to six-word sentences, 100% intelligible

121 On average, a two-year-old has a vocabulary of 50–200 words (see table). Speech is approximately 50% intelligible. These children should by now be using two-word combinations.

122 i. Long-term use of steroids may have substantial undesirable side-effects. The most common adverse effect is suppression of linear growth. Posterior subcapsular cataracts may develop. Other untoward effects include osteoporosis (vertebral collapse), hypertension, diabetes mellitus, cushingoid habitus, infections, pancreatitis, gastritis, and myopathy.
ii. Chronic lung disease becomes a troubling condition to manage long term because of the increased susceptibility these children have to infections. Their steroid use predisposes them to infection, and illnesses require the steroid doses to be increased.

123 i. This child has cellulitis of the gastrostomy site, a diffuse, acute inflammation with hyperemia, edema, and leukocytic infiltration with little or no necrosis. With some organisms, this is followed by necrosis, liquefication, and accumulation of leukocytes and debris; supporation, and formation of one or more abscesses. Infection may spread, leading to bacteremia, septic embolization, and systemic dissemination of infection.
ii. Localized infection can develop in any region of the body, but may be initiated by trauma and secondary bacterial contamination.
iii. Protection of the gastrostomy site with either netting or an enclosed t-shirt as this child is wearing is helpful. The tube should be secured and firmly anchored to prevent irritation from movement. Routine gastrostomy site care with site inspection is crucial. Half-strength peroxide is used initially after insertion; thereafter, soap and water to the site is all that is necessary.

Index

Index

Index